7 SUMMITS

A NURSE'S QUEST TO CONQUER MOUNTAINEERING AND LIFE

DISCARD

PATRICK HICKEY, DRPH, RN, CNOR

College of Nursing
University of South Carolina
Columbia, South Carolina

JONES AND BARTLETT PUBLISHERS

Sudbury, Massachusetts

BOSTON   TORONTO   LONDON   SINGAPORE

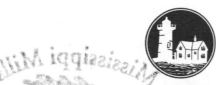

World Headquarters
Jones and Bartlett Publishers
40 Tall Pine Drive
Sudbury, MA 01776
978-443-5000
info@jbpub.com
www.jbpub.com

Jones and Bartlett Publishers
Canada
6339 Ormindale Way
Mississauga, Ontario L5V 1J2
Canada

Jones and Bartlett Publishers
International
Barb House, Barb Mews
London W6 7PA
United Kingdom

Jones and Bartlett's books and products are available through most bookstores and online booksellers. To contact Jones and Bartlett Publishers directly, call 800-832-0034, fax 978-443-8000, or visit our website www.jbpub.com.

Substantial discounts on bulk quantities of Jones and Bartlett's publications are available to corporations, professional associations, and other qualified organizations. For details and specific discount information, contact the special sales department at Jones and Bartlett via the above contact information or send an email to specialsales@jbpub.com.

The authors, editor, and publisher have made every effort to provide accurate information. However, they are not responsible for errors, omissions, or for any outcomes related to the use of the contents of this book and take no responsibility for the use of the products and procedures described. Treatments and side effects described in this book may not be applicable to all people; likewise, some people may require a dose or experience a side effect that is not described herein. Drugs and medical devices are discussed that may have limited availability controlled by the Food and Drug Administration (FDA) for use only in a research study or clinical trial. Research, clinical practice, and government regulations often change the accepted standard in this field. When consideration is being given to use of any drug in the clinical setting, the health care provider or reader is responsible for determining FDA status of the drug, reading the package insert, and reviewing prescribing information for the most up-to-date recommendations on dose, precautions, and contraindications, and determining the appropriate usage for the product. This is especially important in the case of drugs that are new or seldom used.

Production Credits
Publisher: Kevin Sullivan
Acquisitions Editor: Emily Ekle
Acquisitions Editor: Amy Sibley
Associate Editor: Patricia Donnelly
Editorial Assistant: Rachel Shuster
Associate Production Editor: Katie Spiegel
Senior Marketing Manager: Barb Bartoszek

V.P., Manufacturing and Inventory Control:
   Therese Connell
Composition: Shawn Girsberger
Cover Design: Kristin E. Parker
Cover Image: © Patrick Hickey
Printing and Binding: Malloy, Inc.
Cover Printing: Malloy, Inc.

Library of Congress Cataloging-in-Publication Data
Hickey, Patrick, 1955-
  7 summits : a nurse's quest to conquer mountaineering and life / Patrick Hickey.
     p. ; cm.
  Includes bibliographical references.
  ISBN 978-0-7637-7263-5
  1. Hickey, Patrick, 1955- 2. Nurses—United States—Biography. 3. Mountaineers—United States—Biography. I. Title. II. Title: Seven summits.
  [DNLM: 1. Hickey, Patrick, 1955- 2. Nurses—United States—Personal Narratives. 3. Motivation—United States. 4. Mountaineering—United States—Personal Narratives. 5. Nursing—United States—Personal Narratives. WZ 100 H6249 2010]
  RT37.H32 2010
  610.73092—dc22
  [B]
                                          2009002217
6048

BIOGRAPH
796.522

Mississippi Mills
Public Library

Printed in the United States of America
13 12 11 10 09   10 9 8 7 6 5 4 3 2 1

Dedication

To our present and future nursing heroes of health care,
may you all be the patient advocates that our public so desperately needs.

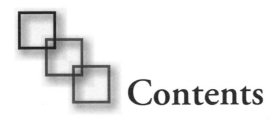

Contents

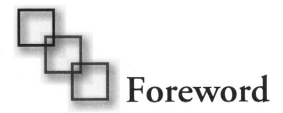

Foreword

In his poem "O Me, O Life," Walt Whitman speaks of every human's opportunity to touch the world. This opportunity is realized by millions of nurses each day through the care that they provide. Nursing care changes the future not only for their patients but for their patients' spouses, children, and future generations as well. The power of nursing rests in the fact that in every act and encounter of nursing there is an opportunity for the nurse to do great good or great harm. This is true for nurses who practice in a clinical role, a leadership role, or an educational role. Each nurse has the responsibility to care for those in his or her charge and each nurse has the power to make his or her mark on the world through the nursing he or she provides. Practicing the art of nursing is truly an adventure and, like the 7 Summits, each opportunity to nurse is a new and unique adventure that must be accomplished carefully.

Pat Hickey has taken the spirit of adventurous nursing to a new level in his quest to elevate his profession. Ever the educator, Pat sees the connection between the challenges of the mountain and the challenges of educating patients and student nurses. He teaches while he climbs so the world might be a slightly better place. His book, *7 Summits: A Nurse's Quest to Conquer Mountaineering and Life*, is a story dedicated to helping young men and women entering the nursing profession.

Pat's quest to conquer the 7 Summits is an amazing story filled with high risk and personal satisfaction. It is not a quest of wealth but of personal measurement and of opportunity to ensure a strong future for the profession of nursing. I hope you enjoy joining Pat on his adventures to the eight highest points in the world—the 7 mountain tops and the classroom full of nursing students.

William Duffy, RN, MJ, CNOR
Vice President of Nursing, NorthShore University HealthSystem
Former President, AORN (2004–2005)

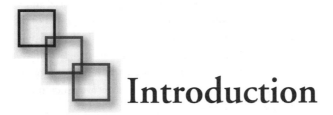

Introduction

I want to share a dream with you. A dream so daring that to act upon it conjures thoughts of lunacy and extreme daring. A dream so wild and fanciful that few have dreamed it, and even fewer have experienced it. A dream that offers an opportunity for tremendous insight through trial in brutally exposing situations, and yet offers a view into the true soul of nature, in all its beauty, temper, and might. A dream in which fears are overcome, and triumph follows the most desperate of outlooks. This dream is my dream, and at times it gives way to peaceful sleep, yet at other times it pushes sleep away as my mind traces the routes, the probabilities, and the challenges.

Most of us dream, and these dreams are usually fanciful thoughts of travel, adventure, and places and people unknown. However, usually those dreams are just that—dreams—a safe haven for exploring the roads less traveled, the paths less trodden, and places unknown. My dream was not only to see the world, but to stand on top of it by climbing to the top of the 7 Summits of the World, which are the highest mountains on each of the 7 continents of the world. A dream that bordered on a high level of fear, teetered across the line of survival, and pushed perilously close to the edge of disaster. I believe that each of us has a sense of adventure within us, yet we are all different in how we exhibit those tendencies. My adventuresome exploits are just more noticeable because they are a little extreme. For some, the adventurer within can compel a person to climb a mountain, run a marathon, learn a new language, travel to a foreign country, or even seek a more challenging job or position of leadership within an organization.

I like to share my adventures with the students I teach, because I know that most will never see the places that I have seen, or do the things that I have done. I recently read an article that described various teaching styles and was pleasantly surprised to see my category was listed: that of storyteller. I have been a storyteller all my life and am sure those stories started as dreams of faraway places, which eventually became reality as I traveled the world and started mountain climbing. Good stories can be very powerful and moving, especially when they include an emotional component. Telling an entertaining story is important, but bringing that personal component to the story makes it much better. In my role as Clinical Assistant Professor in the College of Nursing at the University of South Carolina I believe that reinforcing who I am, through the stories that I tell, not only creates credibility but also helps students to see my passion and creativity. It has been my experience that once students have a memorable story to help them remember a key theme or piece of information, they are much more capable of recalling that information when needed.

While on **Mt. Everest** I shared my stories of an adventurous life, the joys of nursing, and the challenges of mountain climbing through a daily blog. Through use of a satellite phone, a palm-held PDA, a fold-out keyboard, and a variety of adapters and cables, I was able to write my blog, interacting with over 500 people from 20 countries. Those who sent e-mails did so with a sense of curiosity, and always with warm greetings and encouragement. Those words of encouragement got me up the mountain, and I am forever in debt to friends and strangers around the world for their kindness and help when it was needed most. I have included in this book many portions of these blogs, as well as many quotes: all that were sent to me during my 2-month climb up and down **Mt. Everest**. The stories at the beginning of each chapter are those that I have collected over the Internet from fellow climbers and nurses around the world because they, too, carry very powerful messages. Everyone who dialogued with me learned of the challenges in nursing, the nursing shortage, issues with retention, but, most important, they learned of the challenges that face student nurses. Estimates are that at least 40,000 students were turned away from admission to nursing schools last year due to lack of faculty, and those who were accepted were challenged by higher costs of education and a very competitive scholastic environment. As a professor I have seen my student nurses working sometimes up to two and three jobs just to get by, and this added pressure has resulted in increased absences from classes.

Many solutions have been implemented to help abate the nursing shortage, but nowhere near enough. I decided to initiate my own, and just prior to leaving to climb **Mt. Everest** I developed the Summit Scholarship. This scholarship is intended for student nurses at the University of South Carolina College of Nursing, and my goal is to raise $1.00 for every foot of altitude of **Mt. Everest**, which would be a total of $29,035. Plans are to continue developing future scholarships at the national level with proceeds from both this book and the motivational talks that I do around the country. When I stood on top of **Mt. Everest** on May 24, 2007, I became the first nurse in the world to complete the 7 Summits of the World, and I joined an elite group of a little over 100 people in the world who have completed this same journey. I have made it my life quest to take advantage of my "15 minutes of fame" to advocate for nurses by educating the public on how they can contribute to our success by supporting scholarships for nurses.

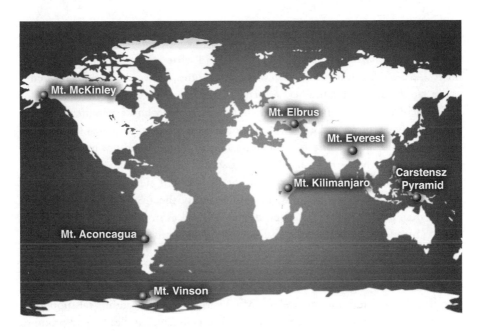

Source: Modified from oblong1/ShutterStock, Inc.

I am adamant that it is the skills acquired as a nurse that have enabled me the opportunity to not only travel throughout 57 countries around the world, but to also stand on top of the 7 Summits of the World. Since graduation with my Nursing Diploma from St. Lawrence College in Brockville, Ontario, Canada, in 1976, I have led a very rewarding life as a nurse. My experiences have been many, triumphs plentiful, and sorrows way too many as I have dealt with a lifetime of pain, death, and dying. My broad range of work experience has included roles as staff, manager, educator, and director, and my workplace settings have ranged from medical-surgical to emergency, surgery, performance improvement, and finally risk management. Professionally, I have been very involved at the local, state, and national levels with the Association of periOperative Registered Nurses (AORN) and owe them a debt of gratitude for helping in my growth as a leader. Additionally, I have been involved at the local and state levels with the South Carolina Nurses Association (SCNA) as well as my local chapter of Sigma Theta Tau.

Through involvement in these roles, committees, and organizations, my communication and cultural competency skills as a nurse have been enhanced, and this growth has helped me immensely when traveling in developing countries around the world; my leadership and team member skills have helped me be a better team player while climbing; my ability to look at the bigger picture from a holistic standpoint has helped me in all venues; and my profession as a nurse has been greeted with great respect from climbers and nonclimbers around the world.

So what? Why should you read this book, and what are the benefits of the book for you? I can tell you that as a result of my adventures, I have changed for the better as a person, a husband, a brother, a teacher, and a son. However, I did so after a lot of heartache on the mountains: from dealing with friends who were injured to others who were dying, prolonged exposure to extreme weather conditions that have left me with numb and tingling fingers and toes for months on end, and not to mention the anniversaries, birthdays, and all of the other special daily events that I missed while climbing up and down the 7 Summits of the World. The support of my wife Carol was most instrumental in not only my completion of the 7 Summits of the World, but in attaining my higher education degrees, as well as in achieving success within nursing organizations. Without her support and love, I would not have been able to accomplish a fraction of what I have done. In addition to the support of my wife I have to acknowledge the support of family, friends, fellow faculty, nursing colleagues, and of course my nursing students in the College of Nursing at the University of South Carolina. During my summit week on **Mt. Everest** I had the additional support of total strangers around the world as many prayers were sent, candles lit, and promises made to get me up and down the mountain safely.

Looking back on my 7-year quest to climb the 7 Summits of the World I wouldn't change a thing, other than to have gotten to know some of my fellow climbers a little better. Of course it would have been great to have my wife Carol climbing with me on all of the mountains, but she discovered her limitations on **Mt. Kilimanjaro** in Tanzania, and to test fate with future climbs at altitude could have been a death wish. My hope is that by reading this book you don't have to go to these extremes to realize the values of life. Don't get me wrong, though: prior to my quest to climb the 7 Summits of the World I had a very healthy outlook on life. But since my final summit I have looked at life differently as framed by my 7 Summits of Life.

To make drastic changes in your life, to live healthier and happier, you don't have to challenge yourself as I have done by climbing the highest mountain on each continent of the world, backpacking through 57 countries around the world, and returning to school during midlife to obtain two master's degrees and a doctoral degree. You don't have to, but if you want to do so, I encourage you to do your research well and make sure that you have a support system that will be there for you, as I did, when you are in greatest need. If you don't want to pursue these physical and mental challenges as I did, you can still make major changes in your life by looking at life as I do now through the 7 Summits of Life, which for me have been the 7 summits of success.

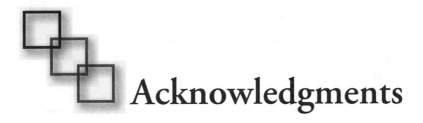

Acknowledgments

I often share my concern that we spend way too much time "writing people up" for having done something wrong and not enough time "catching people doing good things." Now I have the opportunity to walk the walk instead of talking the talk. But where to begin, and whom to note? The pages of my book are filled with those that have helped me in life and range from family and friends to teachers, colleagues, and organizations. Without them I would not have been able to accomplish even half of what I have done.

Upon reflection, a very solid foundation of love and support from family and friends helped me flourish. As I will note later in the text, my brothers and I have adopted our drive and work ethic from our dad and out compassion to help anyone and everyone from our mom. Without these solid roots in our family tree we would not have been able to blossom.

My thanks go out to many colleagues who have supported my efforts to advocate for nursing, and to those people I owe a debt of gratitude. Bill Duffy and Paula Graling have been mentors and friends in perioperative nursing and have done more for me than they will ever know. I can only hope that I can also mentor and inspire others, as they have me; if it were not for their early influence on my nursing career I would not have the skill sets that have empowered me to create change. Dean Hewlett in the College of Nursing at the University of South Carolina has been a staunch advocate for nursing rights and has instilled within me the desire and passion to continue my efforts to create more scholarships for nursing and to challenge my students to be the best that they can be.

I would be remiss if I did not thank those family, friends, students, colleagues, and total strangers—who eventually became friends—who joined me on my blog for a 2-month journey up and down the highest mountain in the world, **Mt. Everest**. On that journey I enjoyed the compassion, friendship, love, and support of well over 500 people from more than 20 countries around the world. In my deepest, darkest moments of despair, when I was freezing to death, hypoxic, hypothermic, and malnourished, these individuals' prayers and well wishes gave me the momentum to continue forward. That investment in my well-being was not in vain, because I have made it my life quest to advocate for nursing and student nurses. A few of those individuals who were staunch supporters were Sandra Dickson, a nursing colleague at Palmetto Health Richland Hospital in Columbia, SC, my best friend, Dr. David Gray, who helped me work through medical dilemmas while on the mountain, and Bonnie Denholm, a perioperative colleague and friend employed by the Association of periOperative Registered Nurses (AORN), whose daily contributions on the blog kept me connected with the "real world." Mary Claire Reinhardt, or MC, was a total stranger during my climb, but I now count her as a friend. You will see MC's quotes throughout my book, and I have to admit that they were inspiring and always came along when I needed them. As you read the excerpts from my blog throughout this book, try to imagine how powerful and motivating these words were to me as I faced the biggest challenge of my life. These same sentiments are just as powerful in our daily lives as we struggle to get up and down our own Everests, so please try to encourage, mentor, and support those around you as often as you can. You may never know that the few words of praise or a simple smile of encouragement could make the difference between life and death.

I keep a folder in my file cabinet at work that contains the cards, notes, and letters of praise and support that I have received over the years from students, colleagues, patients, and those that have attended my presentations. This collective grouping of seemingly inconspicuous pieces of paper is more powerful than the biggest raise one could ever receive and can easily change a mood of despair to one of hope and promise. If it were a pill I'd take it daily and copiously, because the euphoria associated with love, belonging, and support speaks to the basics of our existence. I strongly encourage all nursing students, nurses, and all individuals to create your own "pick-me-up" folder, because more often than not they help you get through the day. A recent addition to my folder is as follows:

> *I wanted to write this email after grades were posted so that you would know that I am being sincere. I just wanted to let you know how much you have made me fall in love with nursing. I originally applied to the university as a criminology major because I thought that was what I always wanted to do. I changed my major after taking an anatomy class my second semester of my senior year. I was not sure if nursing was what I wanted to do but I thought I would give it a try. After taking your class I am sure that I want to be a nurse. Being able to shadow in the labor and delivery department was one of the best opportunities and I just wanted to let you know how much I enjoyed it. Thanks for teaching me about nursing and being so in love with it that it's infectious.*

The friendships that I have developed through international travel and while climbing on mountains all over the world are friendships for life. Many people will come in and out of our lives, but the special bonds that flourish with those that share a passion for life, travel, and adventure are especially strong. When encountering fellow backpackers in a developing country where English is not spoken, or clinging to the side of a mountain roped to a fellow climber that you met only days earlier, there is a tendency to "cut to the chase" and get to know each other at a more primal level, because life and survival are the primary goals. I owe a debt of gratitude not only to my fellow climbers, but also to my guides throughout the years. They have been the reassuring factor as I dealt with the fear of the unknown. The guides at Mountain Trip based out of Ophir, Colorado have become great friends, because they were there with me for four of the 7 Summits of the World. On my last climb of the 7 Summits, **Mt. Everest**, our group came together as team members and friends to make certain that we all accomplished our goal: "Kiwi" Mike Allsop, an Air New Zealand pilot; Bob Jen, a real estate tycoon from New York City; Bo Parfet, an entrepreneur from Michigan (who has written his own book on the trials and tribulations of mountain climbing); Ward Supplee, a carpenter and devoted husband and father from California; as well as Dr. Anna Shekhdar and Dr. Rob Casserley, and Mike Davey, a healthcare analyst, all from Great Britain. To each of these team members I send heartfelt thanks; each and every one of you helped me get to the top of the world. We will always share this sense of pride and accomplishment when our lives changed forever on that triumphant day in May 2007.

And last, but not least, I want to thank my wife Carol for her undying love and support. Without her none of this would have been possible. Throughout my years of mountain climbing she has endured the challenges of communication across the 7 continents of the world and my absence at many of those routine yet invaluable life events, and I am sure that she passed many nights of despair wondering whether or not I would return from the mountains safely. I am eternally grateful for that support, love, and friendship and have no plans to challenge Carol anymore with any death defying dreams. *(In November of 2008 we took our relationship to a new high as we did parallel tandem skydives from 14,000 feet.)*

Never say never…

The photograph on page 64 has been provided courtesy of Alan Arnette. Alan makes his home in Colorado and is an avid climber. He has been a visitor to some of the highest mountains in the world and uses his recognition through climbing to raise funds and awareness for Cure Alzheimer's Disease and to support the Alzheimer's Fund. More information about Alan and climbing can be found at www.alanarnette.com.

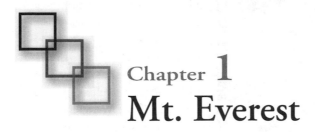

Chapter 1
Mt. Everest

ADVERSITY

Adversity is an unwelcome companion who travels life's road with us.
He is a bothersome fellow bringing sorrow, heartache, and pain.
The heavy burdens that he asks us to carry are his traveling companions.
We take shortcuts and sideroads in hopes of escaping him,
In hopes of a brief reprieve.
But when we turn a corner, there he is again with arms open wide,
Waiting to embrace us.
It seems we cannot escape him!
What to do? What to do?
Let's take his hand and call him friend,
For though he brings turmoil
When he takes his leave,
There is knowledge, strength and purpose left behind,
A clearer vision to see the road that lies ahead.
He allows us to look back and learn from the past
So that we may reach forward to embrace a future of endless possibilities.

—ANONYMOUS

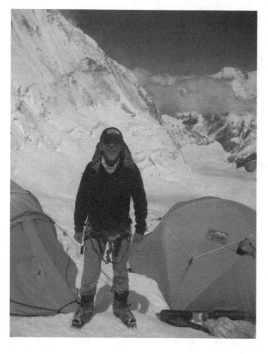

Sunrise at almost 24,000 feet in Camp 3 on **Mt. Everest** was stunning—both the view and the altitude were breathtaking! Was this really happening? Was it a dream, or a nightmare? After 7 years of planning and successful summits of six of the 7 highest mountains on each of the continents of the world, I was now within view of my final summit, **Mt. Everest**. The route to the top from Camp 3 looked more frightening than anything that I had ever seen before because there appeared to be no relief from the extreme angles of ascent that I had already experienced on the lower half of the mountain. With the rise of the sun came an immediate change in temperature as our tent began to bake in the early morning sun. In our haste to move up the mountain, we again failed to replenish our fluids adequately, so we started this next phase of our climb with less than optimal hydration. We also started the climb in down suits because the route ahead was supposed to be cold, and we headed out carrying oxygen for the first time. Additionally, prior to departure, we noted that my regulator might not be accurate, and I was concerned about a possible leak in my oxygen supply. The climb out of Camp 3 starts with the ascent of a 30-foot wall, and by the time I got to the top of the wall I was sweating profusely. At sea level I could have scampered up, but at this altitude I felt like I had hundreds of pounds of bricks in my backpack. It wasn't as cold as expected, and I felt that I had way too many clothes on. I normally overheat easily and usually can tolerate the cold quite well, so I decided to take off my outer layer, which was the high-altitude down suit. It was at this time that members of our extended team, on their way down from Camp 4, stopped to replace my oxygen tank/regulator so that I wouldn't have to worry about a leak.

MyEverest Quote

"Look up, look waaaaay up!"—The Friendly Giant

Putting My Best Foot Forward

Now I was ready to climb, because I was cooler and had a good working oxygen system, or so I thought. However, the sun seemed to focus its burning rays on me alone, and I soon began to dehydrate rapidly. As I climbed the infamous Yellow Band, a yellow striation of bare rock, I noticeably started to slow down, and the wind began to blow stronger. I resisted adding layers of clothing because I felt I could keep warm enough by moving forward. As I slowly climbed the slope up the Geneva Spur, I began to notice the bite of the wind more on my legs, which were covered only by a pair of expedition-weight long johns. The acute angle of the climb at this point brought back my fear of heights, and my forward motion slowed to a crawl as I tried to deal with the extreme drop-off on my left. I hate my fear of heights because it causes all kinds of problems. Because of my fear, I normally slow to a snail's pace as I take extra time to make certain my feet are where they are supposed to be and constantly try to avoid looking at the open, exposed areas all around me. My wife Carol has said that I look like an old man when this happens. I adopt a shuffling movement and at times have been known to get down on my hands and knees on the sides of cliffs or trails when I was most afraid. I also usually develop tunnel vision and feel like I have blinders in place that prevent me from looking left or right.

MyEverest Blog

I am thinking of you as I hear Sting via Police song—"Every move you make, every step you take... I'll be watching you"—the lyrics are out of context a bit as the rock and roll version may take it elsewhere—but for our purposes we are all with you with every step and you have the universal Spirit watching and guiding you with every move you make. Here's to your mission and your continued dialogue with the mountain.—BD

While I was dealing with my fear of heights and trying to manage the steep grade of the Geneva Spur, my oxygen cylinder silently emptied the last few molecules of its contents into my mask, the last oxygen I would breathe until I reached Camp 4 over an hour later. The struggle up and over the peak of the Geneva Spur (at nearly 26,000 feet) seemed prolonged and more difficult and was much more complicated than I thought it should be. Once over it, I was blasted by the winds that swoop down on the South Col. Blowing snow obliterated my route, and I had to consistently halt my forward progress for fear of walking off the narrow trail. Despite the sharp drop in temperature, I still hesitated to add more layers because I kept thinking Camp 4 was just around the next bend. But it never was, and I was getting colder and colder by the minute.

MyEverest Blog

People from all over this world are wishing you success to the summit and back and above all a safe journey. We are with you in spirit! You are on your way!—MC

I finally made the decision to don more clothes but soon realized that I was fighting a losing battle. I tried and tried and tried to put on my down jacket and pants, but ended up wasting way too much time and energy because the wind kept trying to rip the clothes out of my weakened grip. I was rapidly getting hypothermic, and my sense of urgency turned to panic as I suddenly realized that I was in dire straits. As an operating room nurse, I had studied hypothermia because many of our patients required warming after surgery. Hypothermia occurs when the core body temperature drops significantly below normal. Symptoms are categorized into three stages. At Stage I, mild to moderate shivering occurs, hands become numb, and breathing becomes quick and shallow. At Stage II, the pace becomes erratic, stumbling occurs, shivering is violent, and mild confusion begins to set in. At Stage III, difficulty in speaking occurs, there is complete loss of muscle control, and shivering ceases. This typically leads to death. My body was now convulsing so forcibly from the cold that I had to grit my teeth to keep them from fracturing. I was at slightly over 26,000 feet after having just climbed up and over the Geneva Spur, had been without oxygen for about an hour, was still greatly underdressed, and was now feeling the cumulative effects of lack of nutrition, hydration, and sleep. I started stumbling and felt the wind spinning me around. My legs were numb, and I was weak. My pace had slowed to a crawl. Vivid thoughts of my family, wife, and close friends at work flooded my consciousness. Was this what it was like at the end? Where was Camp 4? How much farther did I have to go? Would anyone hear me if I started to scream?

MyEverest Blog

KIA KAHA … Maori language from New Zealand and literally means "Be Strong."—MB

Awareness of Strengths

Moments later, in what felt like an eternity, a yellow spot ahead of me that I had mistaken for a large rock slowly revealed itself as a tent. My emotions overtook me, and I cried with joy for survival and the chance to see my wife again. I thanked God, I sent silent messages to my wife, and I made many promises in return for another chance to live. This place that I had visited in my mind had been very dark and scary, but, paradoxically, it was also calming. My fear of impending death had been counterbalanced by loving thoughts of friends and family. I did not want to die, but if I had, my last thoughts would have been of those who meant the most to me.

However, my challenge was not over; I still needed to make it to the tent. I could see that the wind was trying to rip it off the mountain, but it stood fast and invited me to move forward. I saw other tents, which told me I was entering Camp 4, but no one was outside because the winds were blowing at least 50–60 mph. I stumbled up to the first tent and tried to yell for help, but no words came from my mouth, only unintelligible grunting sounds like those of an animal. No one answered, or at least I could not hear anyone if they did. I tried to stand to walk to the next tent, but my leg muscles would not work. I tried to will my legs to move, but they would not respond. I could still feel them, but they were almost numb. My arms still worked, so I half-crawled to the next tent as I dug my fingers into the ice and snow and pulled myself forward with what little strength I had left. I tried to yell again, but only strange noises came out of my mouth. What was happening to me? Why could I not speak? Why could I not walk?

I was desperate to get out of the weather, so I strained as hard as I could to unzip the outer tent door and as I did, the inner layer door opened and two big arms reached up and pulled me into the tent. I was in the arms of my tent-mates, who had been worried sick about me. At first, I could only grunt a deep primal sound. It took a concentrated, forceful effort with all my being to finally make an intelligible noise. My words were barely audible as I kept mumbling that I was okay, but my two friends knew differently as they worked to warm me up. They had quickly realized the severity of my situation. While one wrapped me in a down sleeping bag, the other placed high-flow oxygen on my face. They removed my boots and outer clothes and vigorously rubbed my extremities to stimulate circulation in the areas most affected by my exposure to the elements. A guide from one of our teams was called in to assess the situation and recommended that three liters of fluids be forced into me ASAP, because we had to depart for the summit within three hours. I remember him questioning whether I was going to be able to leave for the summit in my present condition. I tried to speak in my defense and tried to get up to move about and show that I was okay, but was told to rest, hydrate, and keep warm. Within minutes, I sank into a deep sleep and blocked out the scenario unfolding in front of me.

> **MyEverest Quote**
>
> **"All the adversity I've had in my life, all my troubles and obstacles, have strengthened me... You may not realize it when it happens, but a kick in the teeth may be the best thing in the world for you."**—Walt Disney

When Is Risk Worth It?

I awoke two hours later and felt numb. Where was I? What had happened? What was wrong with me? It was a strange awakening that I will never forget. And the worst part was that I had only 1 hour more to rest before I had to leave the tent to climb to the top of the world, a trek that would take all night long. What had I gotten myself into? Climbing from Camp 4 to the summit was not looking like much of an option because I was still exhausted from the previous climb and had not recovered from my near-death experience. From somewhere outside our tent, a voice yelled out to get ready for a 9:00 PM departure into a night that I had been anticipating, but now did not want. Clothes needed to be layered, fluids and nutrition gathered, hand warmers activated, and skin protection lotions applied. As we went about our preparations, my mind wandered to the task ahead. Was I ready to do this? Had I recovered adequately from the exhaustion of the trip from Camp 3 to Camp 4? Did I have the strength to move onward and upward all night long? What if I backed out now? Would I have another chance to go for the summit? The nurse in me said that this was a mistake waiting to happen; however, I was caught up in the emotion of the moment and moved forward despite the danger. The hour flew by as we methodically moved about our tent in slow motion: dressing, packing, and trying to conserve as much energy as possible.

> **MyEverest Quote**
>
> **"The difference between a successful person and others is not a lack of strength, not a lack of knowledge, but rather a lack of will."**—Vince Lombardi

Standing on top of **Mt. Everest** had been a dream, both frightening and exciting, since 1996. It was during the spring of that year that I first heard of the infamous tragedy of the death of 12 climbers on **Mt. Everest** from Jon Krakauer's book *Into Thin Air.* As a "newbie" to mountain climbing at that time, I felt the anguish of the climbing community; as a nurse, I mourned for their families. Lives taken too early, families destroyed, and legends made. This mountain had been a killer, again. Why were they there? What had gone wrong? Were they prepared? Could it have been prevented? And now here I was, 11 years later, having my training and skills similarly challenged by the forces of nature as I struggled to survive en route to the summit of the highest mountain in the world, at 29,035 feet.

MyEverest Quote

"Climb the mountains and get their good tidings. Nature's peace will flow into you as sunshine flows into trees. The winds will blow their own freshness into you and the storms their energy, while cares will drop off like autumn leaves."—John Muir

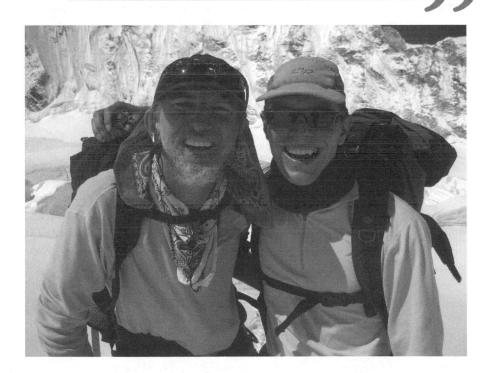

Success Is a Balancing Act

My training grounds for **Mt. Everest** were a variety of volcanoes in Latin America, the Colorado "fourteeners," **Mt. Rainier** in Washington State, and, most importantly, the highest mountains on six of the 7 continents of the world. Along with **Mt. Everest**, these mountains, the "7 Summits of the World," are considered the Holy Grail of mountaineering, because climbing them necessitates that you visit every continent and be challenged with extremes of weather conditions, political unrest, food scarcity, and isolation. Access to these remote mountains is difficult, and costs range in the tens of thousands of dollars because transportation, route finding, and local support can sometimes be more problematic than the actual climb on the mountain. Each mountain has its own particular challenges, but all are physically demanding. Research and planning for each of these mountains resulted in my setting a goal in 2000 to become the first nurse in the world to make it to the summit of each of them. However, this goal was established despite my severe fear of heights, which at times has crippled me on mountain ledges. In 2001, I began my journey, and after climbing one mountain each year for 7 years, I successfully completed my bid to conquer the 7 Summits of the World when I stood atop **Mt. Everest** on May 24, 2007. Though each of the summit bids held risk, adventure, extreme challenges, and fear of death, none compared to **Mt. Everest**. It was the ultimate high, the ultimate risk, and it turned from a pleasant dream into a nightmare that I thought would never end.

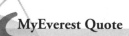

MyEverest Quote

"I didn't conquer Everest—Everest allowed me to crawl up one side and stay on the peak for a few minutes."—Bear Grylls

So many things happened during my climb of **Mt. Everest** that only now, a year after my climb, am I able to collect my thoughts and write those stories down. The summit of the world's tallest mountain was not gained easily, and I felt repercussions from it for several months afterward. Summit Day is the culmination of months and years of training, sheer determination, major willpower, and lots of luck. In my case, it almost never happened for several reasons, including uncontrollable circumstances and challenges that presented themselves at various points along the way. Most obstacles I was able to overcome, but others continued to plague me as I strived to reach the top of the world.

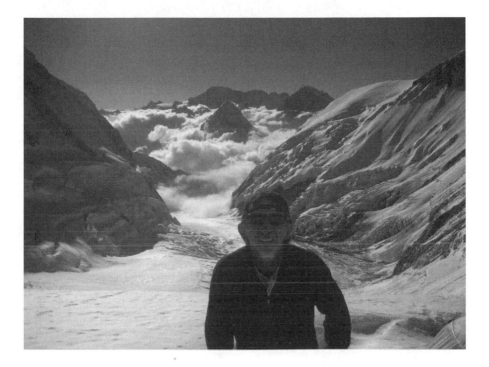

Preparing for the Journey

Your climb to the summit of **Mt. Everest** actually starts several days before Summit Day, and the entire round trip process usually takes a week. You must climb from Base Camp to Camp 1, and then on to Camps 2, 3, and 4, with varying amounts of time spent climbing and resting between each, depending on the weather, your resources, and your level of fitness. But even that amount of climbing only hints at the preparation needed, because, prior to a summit bid, you have already spent almost 2 months training at Base Camp, with repeated forays up and down the mountain between Base Camp and Camps 1, 2, and 3. I didn't realize it at the time, but some of those climbs turned out to be almost too realistic previews of what was to come when I made my bid for real.

My first practice climb from Camp 2 to Camp 3 was harrowing because it was my initial attempt to ascend the Lhotse Face, and unfortunately it was done at midday when I was exposed to the harsh sun at the base of the climb and it followed me all the way up the wall to camp. This climb exhausted me to the point at which I could barely move when I reached camp. With each step, I felt like my legs weighed a thousand pounds, and my heart felt like it was ready to jump out of my chest. Surely everyone must have heard how loud it was pounding because it was deafening to me.

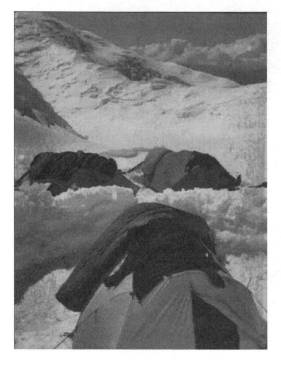

In slow motion, I sat down in my tent, and for the first time, my vision became blurred. I needed water—lots of it, because I knew I was suffering from severe dehydration. But each time I swallowed, it felt like sharp pieces of glass were tumbling through my throat that was so raw from the wind and the heat of the sun.

While trying to recover, I was also rendering first aid and treatment to my tent-mate, Bobby, who was experiencing nausea, severe headache, and abdominal cramps. Bobby was worse off than I was and needed immediate help. I didn't even think about it at the time, but I put someone else's physical complaints ahead of my own, even though I knew we both could be dying because we were above 26,000 feet, the altitude considered the death zone. As a nurse, I had been conditioned to take care of others before myself, but here on the mountain the underlying sentiment was to take care of yourself first or you won't survive! We depended upon the oxygen we carried because this altitude cannot sustain human life, food is problematic because the digestive system is starting to shut down, and there is an increased risk of high-altitude cerebral edema (HACE) and high-altitude pulmonary edema (HAPE). We could not afford to stay long in the death zone because to do so would result in rapid deterioration of all systems, with death as an inevitable result. Fortunately, Bobby and I both recovered and returned a few days later to Base Camp, where we rested again before returning to more practice climbing the next day.

MyEverest Blog

"We may be done for this day but be ready to adapt, improvise, and execute for tomorrow is on its way."—MC

Think Win/Win

A few days before our actual summit bid, our team was split in two for safety reasons and to allow some of the more experienced climbers a bid for the summit. We weren't happy about the split because we were a team, had worked together for the past month and a half, knew each other's strengths and weaknesses, and wanted to summit together. On the day that the "A" team pushed for the summit, those of us on the "B" team woke early and gathered in our mess tent at Base Camp. I entered the tent at about 6:00 AM, excited to hear what progress had been made, only to have my team start laughing at me for no reason. What was wrong? What had I done? Did I dress inappropriately for the occasion? Well, it seems that I did because I was wearing a pair of underwear on the top of my head. Apparently, when I sat up in my tent to finish dressing, a pair of my underwear hanging on my in-tent clothesline decided to deposit itself directly on top of my head. I told everyone that I was just airing out my laundry, but they knew better. It was good for a few laughs and lightened the tone in the tent because all of us had been on pins and needles.

As we drank coffee and waited for our standard breakfast of porridge, toast, and eggs, we listened intently to the occasional crackling of the walkie-talkie radio, which was now the centerpiece of our attention. Garbled words in Nepalese broke the tension: their voices excited, confident, and unafraid. Where were they? How far from the top? What was the weather like? And then it happened. At 7:15 AM, I heard my teammate Bo make his transmission from the top of the world in words I will never forget: "I have run out of road; I guess I'm here." Yay! We all jumped with joy and hugged each other because we were so happy for Bo and so wished that we could be standing there with him. In spirit, we were there together, because we were a team, even though we were separated by 12,000 feet. We soon heard Ward and then Rob as all other members of our team made it safely to the summit of the world. We knew, though, that we could not relax until we saw them again face to face, because the most challenging part of the climb is the way down. Over 80% of the climbers who die on **Mt. Everest** succumb on the descent. If there was ever a time for prayers this was it; we knew the challenges that lay ahead for them. As the day progressed, we nervously drifted in and out of the mess tent for updates on their progress. We were finally able to rest later that day when we heard that they were all safe in Camp 4. They were totally exhausted, but safe.

The Starting Line

That afternoon, we were called in, one by one, to the camp manager's tent. He dictated who went where on the mountain, and when. After a stern speech on safety and challenges outside of our control, we got the message: it was our turn to go, and we would head out the next morning. It was finally here, the challenge that I had been looking forward to for the past 8 years. But was I ready? Would everything be okay? Would we all return? I hated this self-doubt, but I could not prevent it from creeping into my mind. Up until now, I had been so positive and so confident. None of us wanted to show doubt, because it is a sign of weakness and there is no room for weakness at the top of the world. I did my best to push this fleeting thought into the deep recesses of my mind with hopes that it would never return. Now I had to focus: I had supplies to pack, lists to check, and people to notify. Sleep would be very listless tonight.

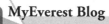

MyEverest Blog

Climbers are driven, high achievers. These people are always doing amazing things. They remind you what an opportunity life is.—MD

Day 1 of the actual summit bid is exhausting because in about 5 hours you climb from Base Camp at 17,500 feet to Camp 1 at 19,500 feet, and after a short rest you face at least another 3 hours to Camp 2 at 21,000 feet, where you spend the first night. The route from Base Camp to Camp 1 is through the infamous Khumbu Icefall, over a treacherous path featuring crevasses, overhanging ice pillars, and 200- to 300-foot ascents and descents. Aluminum ladders are laced throughout the icefall to provide the means to climb over, up, and down the shifting ice that has made this part of the mountain so dangerous. The trail from Camp 1 to Camp 2 has some crevasses marking its otherwise gradual ascent, but it is renowned for the exposure you suffer to the stifling heat of the Western Cwm (*cwm*, pronounced "coom," is Welsh for "valley"). The steepness of the canyon walls and the radiation of intense sun reflected off the snow and the underlying glacier combine to sap your body's fluids until your tongue seems like it is glued to the roof of your mouth. No reprieve from the elements is granted, because to escape the extreme heat of the sun amidst the frigid cold temperatures of the air means a return to Base Camp.

Day 2 is normally a well-deserved rest day at Camp 2, because Day 1 has taken such a heavy toll. The exposure to the heat in the Western Cwm had literally brought me to my knees. While at Camp 2, you try to replenish nourishment, because the higher you climb, the less appetite you have, at a time when you need it most. Cooks try to help by preparing basic meals of rice and vegetables, but taste is lacking and meat is rarely seen.

Day 3 involves climbing from Camp 2 to Camp 3 at 23,500 feet, which can be very challenging because the first few hours are across the Western Cwm and the remaining 3–5 hours are straight up the Lhotse Face—and I mean straight up. It was at the base of the Lhotse Face that the first climber of 2007 was killed when he was struck by ice and rock dislodged from climbers farther up the route. Camp 3 is literally carved out of the side of the Lhotse Face, and the extreme angle requires that you wear crampons on your mountain boots as soon as you leave the tents. Failure to do this has resulted in climbers tumbling 2000 feet into the Western Cwm.

The intense sun at Camp 3 tried to bake us as we lay in our tents, and to cool ourselves we draped our sleeping bags over the top of the tents, but the sun's heat was still intense. In the meantime, we kept the high-altitude stove burning in the foyer of our tent and constantly melted snow, boiling the subsequent water to provide fluids to drink and to cook our meal packets. Hydrate, hydrate, hydrate was my mantra, but the words became empty, because I could never get enough fluids. Focusing on hydration may have been the plan, but it took quite a long time to prepare a measurable quantity of fluids to drink, and Kiwi Mike, my tent-mate, and I were both tired and needed sleep.

Late afternoon turned to evening and as the sun left our tents, the extreme cold set in quickly, the way you feel when a freezer door is opened and you're exposed to its frigid temperatures. With the onset of the cold temperatures, we were less reluctant to get up and gather more snow to melt. Gathering snow was no easy feat, because it required that we put all of our clothing on, including boots and crampons, and leave the tent to dig a sizable amount of snow, place it in a plastic bag, and then carry it back to the tent. It may sound easy, but the simple process of putting on clothes at 23,500 feet is a challenge in itself. Any exertion at all increases heart and respiratory rates that already seem to be competing with each other to see which is faster. Once dressed, you step out into a cold blast of night air that feels as sharp as a knife piercing your lungs. Unfortunately, our laziness and physical weakness made us content with a lot less liquid than what we needed. That night, I did not sleep at all because my mind kept racing to the next night and the knowledge that I would be climbing to the top of the world then. I kept going over the route in my mind, making certain that I maintained all safety measures, kept warm, and made it to the top. I needed sleep *now* to energize myself for the hit that my system would take tomorrow night, but there I lay all night long listening to the steady breathing of my tent-mate, who slept like a log.

Day 4 is a climb from Camp 3 to Camp 4 at 26,300 feet and continues straight up the Lhotse Face to an area called the Yellow Band. This aptly named rock outcropping, crisscrossed with ropes, is unusually challenging because crampons on rock surfaces make for poor grip and slow climbing. After the Yellow Band, the incline becomes much steeper as the route climbs up and over the Geneva Spur, which is not technically challenging but can be very difficult to maneuver depending upon the amount of snow on its surface; if bare, it is very, very dangerous. From the spur, the path is a gradual slope up to Camp 4 on the South Col. Day 4 is extremely challenging because of the sun exposure, and especially because you are using oxygen and carrying a tank for the first time. Once you cross to the South Col, the harsh, biting winds of the jet stream add to the extreme challenge of making it to Camp 4. Normally this trip takes 6–8 hours, but in my case it was an excruciating 12 hours.

Day 5 is the ultimate high: a round trip from Camp 4 to the top of the world at 29,035 feet, and then back again. Summit Day usually starts anywhere from 8:00 PM to 2:00 AM, and it takes you from 12 to 15 hours to reach the summit, and then from 4–8 hours to return to Camp 4. Though it is incredibly thrilling, this day is probably the most exhausting you will ever experience.

Making a Mark That Cannot Be Erased

Summit Day started at 9:00 PM. It was time to go, so we slowly extracted ourselves from the warmth of our tent and found ourselves thrust into a violent windstorm, which dropped the temperature to –10 degrees. In the pitch-black night, faceless voices were barking commands, headlamps were beaming in all directions, and the howling winds added to the confusion. Someone grabbed me, pointed me in the direction where the other headlamps were aimed, and off I walked. Just minutes prior to departure, I met my Sherpa, Dhorjee, and was told that he would accompany me to the summit and back. Sure enough, within minutes "my shadow" fell in behind me on the trail. Dhorjee would maintain that position to the summit of the world, and I quickly became comfortable knowing that he was there for me, should I ever need help. Throughout the night the climb was made more difficult by the blowing snow whipped up by the gale-force winds. Although the skies were clear, and stars could be seen, my view was often obstructed by heavy snow that slapped my face without warning. Our ascent was slowed by the acute angle of the trail, and the pace of the climb was dictated by individual conditioning.

Each of us had our own limitations and could walk only a certain number of steps before we had to stop to catch our breath. No one was pushing us; no one was saying to speed up or slow down. My body told me what to do, but my mind was somewhere else—it was trying to trick my body and convince it that all was well (lotsa luck!). Additionally, we used our Jumar devices to help pull ourselves up the mountain, rhythmically moving the aid to lock and release on the safety line that lay ahead of us. As a nurse, I had been conditioned to use safety lines in the hospital; goggles and gloves were now vital components of patient care, so it was only natural to use these mountaineering aids. Our patterns became repetitive as they had been well rehearsed. In addition to the movement of the Jumar device on the safety line, we would also disconnect and reconnect ourselves to this same line by releasing and then securing a carabiner that connected us by a separate line attached to our harness. Clip in, clip out, clip in became my mantra at the end of each rope and the beginning of the next one. With everyone else, I repeated it up and down the mountain to assure our safety on the fixed ropes. We trudged upward, making sure we stayed connected to the fixed lines. Clip in, clip out, clip in.

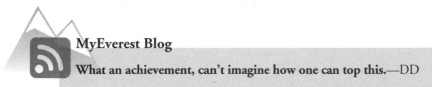

MyEverest Blog

What an achievement, can't imagine how one can top this.—DD

Making Dreams Come True

The first time I managed to look at my watch, it was already 12:30 AM. Wow, we had been climbing for over three hours, and I had not taken a drink of water, nor had I eaten any nourishment! I retrieved a Nalgene bottle from deep inside my down jacket for a long drink of water and devoured half a power bar. I had no time to rest; I needed to keep going. Until then, the only thing I could see clearly was the back of Kiwi Mike in front of me; he was barely within the range of my headlamp. As I looked up the mountain, I could see a parade of headlamps that were climbing as I was, slow and easy. At about 3:00 AM, I started to see the first evidence of light in the east, and I was warmed somewhat by the thought of the coming sunshine; it was something to look forward to in the frigid cold, early hours of the morning.

The "balcony" was a staging area for changing out our oxygen tanks and gave us a moment of rest. We tried to talk while we were there, but our words were muffled by the bulk of our oxygen masks, which resembled those of a fighter-pilot, and the severe winds that howled all around us. Then it was onward and upward. As late night changed to early morning, the rising sun started to give shape to our surroundings, and for the first time I had a glimpse of how exposed we were as we climbed. I say that I had a glimpse because that is all I could manage: I did not want my fear of heights to scare me too much. The worst thing that could happen to me at that time would have been for me to "freeze up" on the side of the mountain out of fear. From that moment on, I purposely avoided looking to my left or right, instead keeping my eyes focused straight ahead on the trail and the safety line. There was no way that I wanted to see how high up I was or how perilous it looked, although I had more than a sneaking suspicion that I was in way over my head.

As I approached the South Summit and the Hillary Step, my pace had slowed noticeably because I was now more aware of my surroundings—and the severe drops in altitude seemed to be everywhere. It appeared that the angle of the mountain was becoming more acute as I climbed higher. I am sure that the altitude helped slow me down somewhat because I was now at close to 29,000 feet, had been climbing steadily for about 12 hours, and was ready for it all to be over. Dhorjee was now urging me to move forward by pushing my back, even though I shuffled my feet along like an old man. And then suddenly, there it was: the summit. I could see my friends at the top and realized it was definitely within my reach, only minutes away. I consciously took my time now because I wanted to enjoy these last few steps to the top of the world.

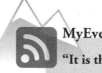

MyEverest Blog

"It is the journey, not the destination."—CP

The actual summit of **Mt. Everest** is small and adorned with hundreds of multi-colored Tibetan prayer flags. There were only a few people ahead of me on the summit, and I was happy to see that all were my friends. I sensed someone near me and turned to see that it was my tent-mate, Mikey. I stepped aside to let him go ahead of me and then slowly followed him to the top. I reached the summit, and after a quick glance over the edge to make sure that there was nowhere else to go, I sat down to try to absorb what I had done.

Top of the World: May 24, 2007, 9:30 AM. Wow! I was finally here after 8 years of planning and 7 years of climbing the highest mountain on each of the 7 continents of the world. I had so many people to thank, and so many things to be thankful for, but first I had to call Carol and let her know I had made it. I dug my satellite phone out of my down jacket, carefully removed my down mittens, and slowly pressed the nearly frozen keypad numbers. It was 9:30 AM, Thursday, on top of **Mt. Everest**, but it was only 11:45 PM the previous day (Wednesday) in Columbia, SC. We connected, and despite 40 mph winds and a temperature of –40, I was able to say, "Carol, I'm here

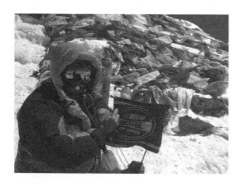

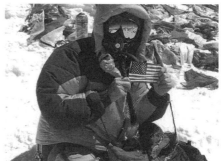

on top of the world, and you are with me. I love you so much." The conversation was short because it was difficult to talk, but the message was clear: I had made it.

MyEverest Blog

Pat just called and reported that he was on the summit (@ 9:30 AM Nepal time). They departed @ 9:30 PM on Wed night. He said it was a beautiful morning but very cold and windy. He couldn't talk much as he was on oxygen and the winds were high. I asked if they had all summitted and he said he thought yes. He said Mikey was there with him. Wendy, I wish I had your number to call you but maybe you will see this post. Pat will be reporting with an audio blog when he returns to Camp 4 or lower. Thanks to everyone for your support & all your well wishes to Pat and me. I'm off to bed for a better sleep than I've had in a few days! Thank you God!—Carol

Running Out of Time

My phone call completed, I decided it was time for photos. I dug deep into my pack again for my digital cameras and offered them to Dhorjee so he could take pictures of me with some of my sponsor regalia. The emotions of the moment caught up with me, and I pulled off my snow goggles to wipe away a tear and was blinded by the sunlight. The flash of light was acutely painful and something I had never experienced before. I quickly refitted my goggles but had to remove them again moments later because of the searing, blinding pain in my eyes. Within a few minutes, I discovered that I could not see out of my right eye, and my left eye had become very blurred. I tried to tell Dhorjee that something had happened to my eyes, but with his limited ability to understand English and the roar from the 40-mph winds, he was unable to understand my frantic gesturing. What had happened? What was going on? Why couldn't I see? Where was everybody? Who could help? All of these questions and more were on my mind, but no one was able to answer me. Within minutes, my joy and exhilaration had turned to sheer terror. All I knew for sure was that I had a major problem, and I was alone on top of the world.

MyEverest Quote

"Courage is resistance to fear; mastery of fear—not absence of fear."—Mark Twain

Getting down from the top of **Mt. Everest** was probably the most difficult thing I have ever done in my life! I thought that getting to the summit would be hard (and it was extremely difficult), but getting off the top was even harder. When I started my descent, I was blind in my right eye, had blurred vision in my left eye, and was concerned that I could not get my Sherpa, Dhorjee, to understand what was happening to me—not that I myself knew. Just minutes off the summit, I caught up with Dhorjee, who had retreated from the top due to the extreme cold! I continued to try to explain to him that I had problems with my vision, but he still did not seem to understand and again walked away from me. He seemed intent on getting down the mountain. I, too, wanted to get down but knew that I would need help.

MyEverest Blog

Be safe, have fun, and remember it all.—BP

And then it happened, at the very top of the world, just below the summit: I fell. My foot had tangled in a rope, and I tripped and fell forward. I remember yelling into my oxygen mask. Although I knew that no one had heard me above the roar of the wind, it was deafening in my ears. Panic, fear, and sheer terror gripped my body as I fell onto the trail in front of me. I lay there motionless, not knowing which way my body was poised to fall: a quick descent into Tibet, 10,000 feet below, or a steeper drop, back into Nepal, 12,000 feet below. Thank God the shortcut to Tibet was a little farther ahead of me, because I fell on a section of the trail that was actually forgiving of a fall. In what seemed like an eternity, Dhorjee arrived and sat me up to see what was wrong. I took advantage of my seated position and removed my snow goggles. He examined my swollen right eye, which was weeping fluid, and my left eye, which was partially open and also weeping. They say a picture is worth a thousand words, and as soon as Dhorjee saw my eyes, it seems like our communication problems were solved. He immediately understood.

MyEverest Quote

"Getting to the summit is optional. Getting back down is mandatory."—Ed Viesturs

Choosing My Destination

I would like to say that the trip down was much easier now that Dhorjee realized I had a problem, but it wasn't. Dhorjee remained very close to me, but I still had to navigate challenging sections of the trail. Soon after my initial fall, I was on the Hillary Step and fell again as I tried to navigate down its face. I found myself dangling in ropes just off the top of the step and after reassurance from Dhorjee was able to make it to the base of the step. My pace continued to be very, very slow because it took so much more effort for me to strain my good eye to see where to put my feet. I was very astute at making certain that I clipped in/out of the safety lines properly because I did not want to risk a fall. Also, we stopped more frequently on the way down because I was starting to feel tired from the lack of sleep, hydration, and nutrition. At the balcony, I shared the last of my fluids with Dhorjee because he had not drunk all evening. We still had a long way to go, and now we set off without fluids. Dhorjee made sure that I had a new oxygen tank, and I think he turned up the oxygen flow to help me get down.

MyEverest Blog

The descent is all the battle.... It doesn't count if you make it up but don't make it down. Be diligent. Boil up as much as possible at camp 4 before the descent. Keep your feet warm and dry. Stay focused. I'm thinking about you guys.—W

Nothing Is Impossible

The trip down to Camp 4 took about 5–6 hours, and I again fell, tripped, and slid a few more times before I arrived safely at camp. Each fall was scarier than the previous, yet I seemed to be getting used to them, and that was even scarier. About halfway down, I noticed that my legs were starting to tremble, and it wasn't from the cold. It seemed like my muscles were wasting away, and they were twitching and cramping uncontrollably. I had experienced this only a few times in my life, and each time was associated with severe exhaustion. As I approached Camp 4, I had little to no control of my legs and felt like a zombie: I would throw one leg out to the side and then the other in order to move forward. It seemed to take forever to get to Camp 4, even though I could see it for hours. On arrival, Camp 4 looked exactly like I had seen it before, with raging winds trying to rip the tents off the mountain. I crawled into my tent and found my teammates fast asleep, and within minutes I, too, was asleep, sitting up, fully clothed.

Discovering Purpose and Passion

Of all the things I have considered since that death-defying trip, my strongest belief is that my **Mt. Everest** summit, and the mountain climbing experiences of my other six summits, has helped me gain a clearer perspective than I have ever known. I see life in general more clearly, and I see quite specifically the 7 things that helped me accomplish this fantastic goal of standing on top of the world: (1) *balance* in life, (2) physical *wellness*, (3) established *goals*, (4) a positive *attitude*, (5) realization of my *potential*, (6) a yearning for *success*, and (7) the opportunity to create a *legacy*. I refer to these specifics as the "7 Summits of Life" in recognition of how each of these attributes has helped me to attain my goals, and I view the 7 summits of my real life as a metaphor for those 7 summits of success in anyone's life.

Moreover, it is important for me to view the 7 Summits of Life through my experience as a nurse, because I feel strongly that it is those skill sets that have prepared me for anything in life—especially climbing the highest mountain on each of the continents of the world, including the highest in the world, **Mt. Everest**. In subsequent chapters, I will expand on these 7 Summits of Life and tell you what I have learned from my experiences during my travels through life, my journey in nursing, and my climbs on the mountains.

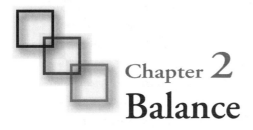

Chapter 2
Balance

Take Hold of Every Moment

A friend of mine opened his wife's underwear drawer and picked up a silk paper wrapped package.

"This," he said, "isn't any ordinary package." He unwrapped the box and stared at both the silk paper and the box.

"She got this the first time we went to New York, 8 or 9 years ago. She has never put it on and was saving it for a special occasion. Well, I guess this is it."

He got near the bed and placed the gift box next to the clothing he was taking to the funeral home. His wife had just died. He turned to me and said: "Never save something for a special occasion. Every day in your life is a special occasion." I still think that those words changed my life. Now, I read more and clean less. I sit on the porch without worrying about anything. I spend more time with my family and less at work. I understood that life should be a source of experience to be lived up to, not survived through. I no longer keep anything. I use crystal glasses every day. I'll wear new clothes to the supermarket if I feel like it. I don't save my special perfume for special occasions. I use it whenever I want to. The words "someday" and "one day" are fading away from my dictionary. If it's worth seeing, listening, or doing, I want to see, listen, or do it now.

I don't know what my friend's wife would have done if she knew she wouldn't be there the next morning; this nobody can tell. I think that she might have called her relatives and closest friends. She might have called old friends to make peace over past quarrels. I'd like to think she would go out for Chinese, her favorite food. It's these small things that I would regret not doing, if I knew my time had come. I would regret it because I would no longer see the friends I would meet, or write the letters that I wanted to write "one of these days." I would regret and feel sad, because I didn't say to my brothers and sons, not enough at least, how much I love them.

Now, I try not to delay, postpone or keep anything that could bring laughter and joy into our lives. And, on each and every morning, I say to myself that this could be a special day, as each day, each hour, and each minute is special.

—Anonymous

What is balance in life, and who or what determines balance? Do we have a scale to indicate when that balance has been reached? And if so, does it also note why one side is out of balance compared to the other, and which factors cause an imbalance to occur? Is my balance in life comparable to others, and is it fair to compare how balanced we are as related to others? At what age in life do we discover balance, and which life experiences help us to become more balanced? As adults, we strive to be the best that we can be to our spouses, children, coworkers, and community; however, to achieve that balance, we must prioritize the amount of time spent at home, at work, at school, in professional organizations, and in our community. Do you really think that on your deathbed you'll wish that you'd spent more time at work? And in the balancing act of deciding what to do first, and how much energy to invest in each endeavor, we also need to be concerned with our financial and health challenges.

My Travels Through Life

MyEverest Quote

"Traveling may be ... an experience we shall always remember, or an experience which, alas, we shall never forget."—J. Gordon

Growing up as the eldest of nine children with one working parent holding down two jobs, hand-me-down clothing as a significant part of my wardrobe, and never any money for movies or pleasantries, did not, at an early age, lend itself to a future of travel and adventure. However, it was my mind that would take me to the four corners of the world, where I imagined I met foreigners dressed in brightly colored flowing robes, uttering languages I could not discern, and eating foods that I had never tasted. In these foreign lands, the people rode bikes on cobbled or dirt streets or paddled hollowed-out tree trunks down churning brown rivers. There was intrigue and adventure around every corner, trouble lurking in every marketplace, and all of this was accompanied by tropical climates, savory smells, and mystical music.

Sharing the Joy

However, something was missing in those daydreams, and that was a travel mate. In all of these imaginary trips to these faraway places, I traveled alone. That changed when I met my future wife Carol, because the two of us were destined to travel the world, together. Since that meeting 25 years ago, we have visited all 7 continents and 57 countries to date. Our itineraries have been at the budget level, using backpacks as our only luggage, accommodations in youth hostels and pensions, and travel on rafts, rickshaws, trains, planes, and automobiles.

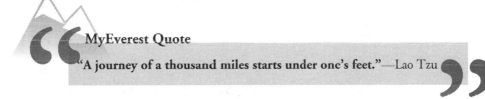

MyEverest Quote

"A journey of a thousand miles starts under one's feet."—Lao Tzu

Travel has given me a balance in life that no classroom education or book ever could. My teachers have been the native inhabitants; my classrooms have been their country. My lessons have been the development of appreciation for the strengths in diversity and the challenges of poverty. The knowledge gained from these lessons I now apply on a daily basis as I work within my community to ease the burden of access to health care, and I translate it into the course for my nursing students. Travel has balanced me as a person because I am much more accepting of people from other countries, and I am more aware of their needs and concerns.

In keeping with the theme of travel and balance, there have been many occasions that I can look back and see where I have not assessed a situation properly and in my attempts to work through an issue have not properly balanced all the facts as I should. One example that stands out occurred during our year of backpacking through Latin

America. It was November 1993, and it had been 11 months since we left our home in Columbia, SC. Our destination was the southernmost tip of South America, Ushuaia, Argentina. We were in Puerto Montt, Chile, and had heard of an exciting and inexpensive boat trip down the coast to Puerto Natales. We decided to join other backpackers on this 4-day journey. However, when we went to purchase tickets we were told that the scheduled ship was being repaired, which left us with two options: we could travel on a smaller ship at a lower fare, or we could wait 2 more days for the regular ship to be back in service. Neither time nor money was an issue for us because we had been traveling very inexpensively and were not restrained by any schedule. However, impatiently, and despite a subtle warning that we might experience a little more wave action in this smaller boat, we decided to go for it. They say that hindsight is 20/20, and when looking back on a situation we see how obvious the problems were at the time.

Well, it seems that in our haste to depart Puerto Montt, we were actually putting our lives at risk but did not know that until a few days later when our boat transitioned from an intracoastal seaway, protected by barrier islands, to the open Pacific Ocean. Our first clue that something was amiss occurred during the middle of a bright, sunny, calm day when the crew started lashing down everything that could move, to walls, doorways, and fixed objects. We initially thought it was some type of joke until we left the protection of the islands, and that's when "all hell broke loose." Our tiny boat started to rock and roll in the huge waves so much that everyone had to scramble to get off the open decks for fear of being tossed overboard. Those who had cabins retired to safety and stayed there for the duration of the trip, whereas those of us with deck tickets moved into the shelter of a forward lounge and hung on to walls, pillars, and each other to avoid tumbling across the room. Anything and everything that had not been tied down shifted with the constant roll of the ship, and we continually had to fend off furniture to prevent being harmed. A putrid odor enveloped the ship because everyone was now throwing up, and in the close quarters the sounds of moaning, groaning, and gagging were deafening. A very loud crash from the rear deck scared all of us more than we already were, and we collectively started to expect the worst—a sinking ship.

Moments later a crewman made his way to the lounge. Despite his years of experience at sea, it was clear that he, too, was very frightened. He motioned to the back of the ship and in a very loud voice told us that an 18-wheeler semitrailer truck had been ripped off the deck. We could not believe what he said, so I scrambled to the back of the boat, slipping and falling all the way—and sure enough, just as the crewman had said, the truck was gone! What made it worse was the swell of the waves, and actually seeing how gigantic they were as they washed across the deck. This was not good.

All that day, throughout the night, and into the next afternoon, we continued to toss and roll, move up and down, and slide left and right. My inner ear was so confused that it took me days to recover and get my "land legs" so that I could walk again.

When we finally passed behind the protection of the barrier islands, the boat settled into a rhythmic calm and seemed to float across the water. People slowly started to reappear, all looking quite haggard, clothes askew, hair jutting in all directions, with a foul smell of puke emanating from our pores. Ironically, it was at that moment when the captain of the ship announced over the loudspeaker that in celebration of this vessel's *first* ocean voyage, there would be free whiskey for all! I don't believe any bottles were opened because we all were still too sick to drink and just felt lucky to be alive.

My Journey in Nursing

I like to think of my profession of nursing as a journey, with an adventurous route, challenging experiences, and an ever-present fear of the unknown. As an immature youth, how prepared was I to take this trip? What life experiences, if any, could I depend on to help me down this unknown trail? And, how did I know if I had chosen the right path?

Balancing Life as a Student Nurse

Through a stroke of fate I was called to nursing. Well, actually, there were many influences and contributing factors, but for the most part it was fate. However, as predetermined as it was, the trail to completion of my degree was wrought with obstacles, detours, and crevasses, and became a personal challenge of the fittest. In order to survive school, as with any mountain climb, there must be a lot of preparation, with the onus of responsibility falling on the student. Planning the route involves good map-reading skills because you need to be able to see what is ahead and prepare accordingly. The various paths to an ADN, diploma, or BSN all end with an RN degree; however, it can be a long journey with many switchbacks in the trail. Once the degree choice is made, the journey begins with base camp as the starting place.

MyEverest Quote

"The mountains have rules. They are harsh rules, but they are there, and if you keep to them you are safe. A mountain is not like men. A mountain is sincere. The weapons to conquer it exist inside you, inside your soul."—Walter Bonatti

Faculty will be the climbing guides for the trip, and their GPS system marks progress through the school curriculum. In the hospital setting, those guides are the clinical educators, CNS nurses, and managers. Some guides will be better than others because experience, communication skills, and work ethic play a major role in how they transfer their knowledge. Make certain that there is a clear vision of where you are going and what you need to get there because many a climb on the mountain, and patient care activity in the hospital, has been aborted due to misunderstandings of expectations. On the mountains, as in the hospital, always be prepared for the worst.

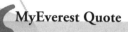

MyEverest Quote

"The day on which one starts out is not the time to start one's preparations."—Nigerian Proverb

Over the years I have listened to the stories of my nursing peers and have always marveled at their abilities to surmount the most difficult of patient care situations, and to do so with ease. I have always wanted to be that nurse who could do it all, who could handle each and every situation, and I have always wondered how long it would take me to get there. But I soon discovered that it would take time and experience. As I began to draw parallels between my life outside the hospital and my profession within it, I found that the challenges I faced as a nurse were very similar to those I experienced when mountain climbing. And then, all of a sudden, everything made sense.

Nursing and Climbing With a View to the Top

In order to increase the chances of a successful venture in school, skills such as organization, study habits, and ability to function as a team member in study groups and the clinical setting need to be adopted and honed. As with any mountaineering trip, there will be a team, and the teammates for this journey will be your fellow classmates. Teammates in the hospital are more diverse and comprised of physicians of all specialties, as well as professionals in radiology, physical therapy, respiratory therapy, and occupational therapy, just to name a few. Each team member brings strengths and weaknesses to the team, yet all contribute to its strength. In mountain climbing men dominate the sport, whereas in nursing it is quite the opposite: men comprise only 5.8% of the nursing population. The average age of a teammate in nursing is about 46 years, whereas in mountain climbing the average age of a mountain/rock climber is 22.7 years.

The gear for the trip through school is not unlike the gear for a mountain climb: the student uniform is like the Gore-Tex outfit of a climber; the stethoscope that we use to auscultate diagnostic sounds is like the headlamp that guides the climber through darkened areas; and the watch that allows us to chart the pulse and respirations of our patients is like the altimeter that climbers use to gauge their position on the mountain.

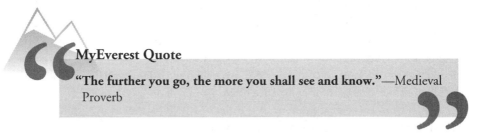

MyEverest Quote

"The further you go, the more you shall see and know."—Medieval Proverb

To further this nursing/mountain climbing analogy, let's start at the beginning. Students start nursing school (base camp), working hard to advance each semester to a higher level of education (strategically placed camps en route up the mountain) to reach the ultimate goal: graduation and the completion of the NCLEX exams (the final push to the mountain summit).

One of the challenges that most students will face on their journey is financial: they will need to work to raise money to pay for school. With this in mind, I developed the Summit Scholarship at the School of Nursing at the University of South Carolina and the Nurses Can Do Anything Scholarship at the National Student Nurse Association, which aim to alleviate this burden somewhat because distractions in school can be just as damaging to your future as distractions on the mountain. I look upon the scholarship as an investment in the future of nursing because these present-day students will be the nurses of tomorrow who will care for us as we age. It is my hope that by establishing scholarships for student nurses, more will attend classes without needing to work, and these caregivers will be up-to-date with all of the latest treatment modalities. Scholarships are available for students; however, there just aren't enough.

Balance in life is very important in adulthood, yet in many ways it is learned in childhood. As a child, my balance was greatly influenced by those around me, and most times, if not all, I was left to discover what worked and what didn't. Some of my earliest memories related to balance involved weighing the options of playing outside longer with my brothers or spending more time on my homework. My decision to go with the rather extended play periods helped me to avoid schoolwork, because school for me then was never easy, caused me great distress, and made me feel like more of an idiot than I already was! Unfortunately, this became a habit with me that grew over time and followed me throughout my experiences as a student. I never learned how to find balance in my personal life, so I neglected my classes. I know today that this lack of balance caused me great challenges in school because I was always ill prepared for class, lacked a depth of knowledge of the subject matter, and never sought additional help. This imbalance led to low passing grades and an ever lower self-esteem as I constantly struggled with almost every class in grade school, high school, and college.

Family, friends, and classmates help to build a support system, as do faculty as mentors. Juggling a job and a full course load can cost grades and health due to lack of sleep and unhealthy eating. Setting aside "me" time—with activities such as working out, taking a long walk, watching a movie, talking to friends, sharing a meal, and shopping—is important for students. Whatever the activity is, it should be for the individual and not related to school or work. Even an hour a day devoted to this activity will help reduce stress and bring balance to life.

Schoolwork aside, what a difference age makes! My imbalance as a youth has transferred to greater balance as an adult. The early developmental challenges that I experienced have helped me in my role as a university nursing professor to better understand my students because I know now that their priorities may be similar to what mine were at that age. As a result of that early imbalance, I am now better prepared to assist my students in finding balance as I help them to prioritize their educational needs.

Balancing Professionalism as a New Nurse

MyEverest Quote

"**Keeping to the main road is easy, but people love to be sidetracked.**"—Lao Tzu

So, as you try to achieve balance, who and what are your support systems? Do you have the support of your healthcare team, your faculty, your family? As a new nurse, I had balance issues again when too many things got in the way of what I wanted to do, and again I had challenges with prioritizing what was more important to me at that time and place in my life. When we are young, we tend to live for the moment with little concern for the future; everything seems to be done for instant gratification. As a relatively new trauma room nurse in southeast Texas, I had to balance acquiring skills to work in a Level 1, fast-paced emergency room; develop an awareness of cultural norms associated with the local Hispanic population; assimilate into a new country somewhat different from my birthplace in Canada; and deal with the death and dying of my patients on an almost daily basis. The fine balance of life and death in these patients triggered within me a desire to be the best that I could be in the emergency room. I remember wishing that I could have done more to help those who died but did not know what to do because I did not have the skills. I found that I was not prepared for the daily challenges of the ER and wanted to bring more to the team. This feeling of helplessness drove my pursuit to take charge of my professional life, so I set the priority of seeking national certification in my specialty, which I felt would bring balance to my life.

As a stepping stone to this end, I became certified in advanced cardiac life support and eventually became an instructor in both basic life support and advanced cardiac life support. With the required years of experience, and some trepidation, I sat for the national exam. It was a very proud day when I was able to add the national designation of certified emergency nurse (CEN) to my name badge. In my mind this national certification, the various levels of instructor status, and years of experience validated for me that I had done as much as I could do to effectively help tilt the balance of the scales of life and death in a more favorable position for my future patients.

Balancing Work-Life as a Nurse

In nursing we have great opportunities to spend a lot of time at work because the need is great and the overtime is plentiful. However, before we choose to work extended periods of overtime we need to evaluate the effects of this overtime on achieving a work-life balance. Fatigue is a critical factor for those nurses working extended periods because it can affect decision-making ability and potentially lead to a mistake. These mistakes could lead to patient safety incidents and negatively affect one's reputation. It is critical to maintain ties with your support system: attending family events—such as birthdays, reunions, and weddings—and spending time with *friends* should not be avoided due to spending too much time at work. If overtime is needed, it should be well planned in order to balance home-life and work-life.

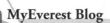

MyEverest Blog

Your passion for nursing and your quest for the summit certainly paves the way to conversations with people interested in a nursing profession. I am not sure people realize the opportunities that nursing provides for people and the difference it makes to patients to have a nursing perspective. Our profession is different from other healthcare professions—may be hard to explain, but we need to keep trying as nurses are a different type of patient advocate and play such an important role in patient safety.—BD

In order to balance work-life, it is crucial to implement some changes into an already hectic routine. One beginning would be to do a needs assessment of sorts by keeping a log of all activities, both work and family related. Once the log is complete, evaluate for issues such as time spent at work, workload, and family time. Prioritization of time and activities conducive to a healthy lifestyle is necessary to balance work-life because too much time in one can cause you to neglect the other. If time at work is an issue, check with your employer to see if there are alternate shifts such as Baylor plans, which allow you to work all weekend with weekdays off, or other options such as flextime, job-sharing, telecommuting, or even part-time employment. Try to avoid working on your day off so you can take care of yourself by adopting an exercise program, setting time aside for family, and getting enough sleep.

Learning to say no to an employer may be hard to do, but it does help keep our lives balanced as we need to consciously not overcommit ourselves to too many events. If workload is an issue, you may need to reevaluate what needs to be done at work and home, and delegate duties as needed. If family time is an issue, explore options such as babysitters, take-out meals, family nights, cooking together, and sharing responsibilities. And finally, use technology to your advantage: cell phones and PDAs can create opportunities to place calls and do work while commuting or attending events.

Assuming leadership roles, combined with the obligations of life, can be overwhelming because we may feel the necessity to get things done and check them off our list. Adding to this challenge are the number of nurses, retention of employees, job satisfaction, and safety issues. These leadership opportunities are choices that we should make to connect and interact with others in our profession, yet are they being done as an opportunity to make a difference, or as an obligation to do something? We need to ask ourselves how we are living our lives because too much multitasking can actually decrease our efficiency and our output.

Burnout has become a common expression associated with overwork and too much stress. In nursing, this can start as early as the student stage. As the director of performance improvement, I used to juggle way too many responsibilities because I felt there was a stigma associated with saying, "I can't do this." Eventually the late hours and heavy workload took its toll and I had to leave that position. I got to the point where I would be the last one left at work, late at night, with no end in sight to the workload.

My Climbs on the Mountains

When most people think of balance, especially on mountains, I am sure that they think of precipitous ledges, death-defying drops, and perilous narrow routes up and down the sides of unforgiving rock and snow covered terrain. All mountains challenge both the physical and mental skills of climbers. So, how does one establish this balance, and just how critical is it to have both a physical and mental balance?

Balancing What Matters Most

MyEverest Blog— Happy National Nurse's Week

Although I'm not a nurse or medical professional [just a mother of 5 working the last 25 yrs in the admin field in the USA], I would NOT want to live in a world without Nurses. Why would one wonder why there are so many nurses/doctors/medics there (on the mountains)? Maybe they like the view; they want to summit Everest; they like to hike on their time off; they feel it's their calling/duty; they can make a lot of money from dummies that fall down the mountain? I DOUBT IT! I bet they are there because they care and they know there is a NEED for them with their knowledge to be there ... be able to help & assist. BECAUSE NURSES CAN DO ANYTHING! This is just what I THINK/BELIEVE & YOU are living proof.—R

On the mountains, there were many occasions when balance in life was an issue. The difference between life and death could be as simple as a snow bridge across the trail, an avalanche descending on a tent, a dramatic change in weather, a lack of supplies or inadequate resources, lack of training, or a medical condition left unchecked. On **Mt. McKinley** in Alaska that fine balance between life and death became a reality when a climber dying from high-altitude cerebral edema (HACE) faced imminent death, with few resources at hand and no one trained to deal with the medical dilemma. It was September 2003, and I had just flown from Talkeetna,

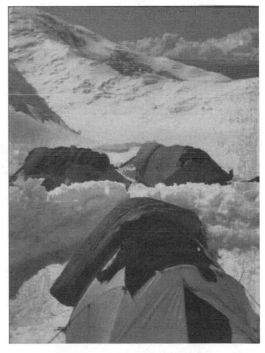

Alaska, onto the Kahiltna Glacier, which is Base Camp for the climb on **Mt. McKinley**. I flew onboard a Cessna 172 that was stripped to the basics to accommodate

enough climbers and gear possible to get it up and over the "one-shot" pass. I can remember seeing the ruins of a recently destroyed plane, just below the pass, that had been hit by a wind shear and crashed into the rock wall. No one survived. The risks in mountain climbing exist not just on the mountains themselves but also on the approach and departure because of the remoteness of these areas.

It was 3:00 AM on our first night at Base Camp when we were woken by our guide. We had planned to break camp early so we could start moving up the mountain. Because we were so far north, we were experiencing midnight sun, which is a phenomenon in which the sun never really sets and daylight hours are experienced all day long and into the night. At this hour, it was bright enough that we could read a newspaper outside our tents. The plan was to move early because the sun would be more intense soon and the snow lower on the mountain would become very slushy and difficult to walk through. As we tore down tents and packed gear, a national park ranger housed at Base Camp approached us. He asked whether there was anyone medical on our team because he needed to start an intravenous (IV) solution on someone. I stepped up immediately and responded that I was a nurse and that I could help start the IV. Our mountain guide was reluctant to have me leave the group because he was intent on departing as soon as possible to avoid poor climbing conditions. I reassured him that I would be back soon after I assessed the situation; but that was not to happen because the situation was drastic.

Putting First Things First

As I entered the three-person tent, I saw a fully clothed climber having what appeared to be a seizure. His involuntary body spasms and thrashing arms and legs jerked his torso free from the sleeping bag that was wrapped around him. I immediately turned to his two climbing mates and asked what had happened. They responded that they had successfully made it to the summit of **Mt. McKinley** earlier that day and when doing so their friend became confused, disoriented, complained of a severe headache, and was nauseous. A doctor at high camp had told them that these were symptoms of HACE and strongly recommended that they descend to the lowest level possible to help his condition. HACE, an extreme, potentially fatal form of altitude illness called acute mountain sickness (AMS), involves swelling of brain tissue due to a very rapid ascent of altitude. Symptoms are usually headache, nausea and vomiting, disturbed gait, loss of consciousness, seizures, coma, and potential death. Treatment normally includes a rapid descent of at least 500 feet, as well as medicines such as dexamethasone.

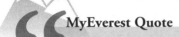

MyEverest Quote

"The art of medicine consists in amusing the patient while nature cures the disease."—Voltaire

According to the group, they had descended as rapidly as possible and had actually made record time getting to Base Camp. However, their friend had continued to feel ill, and when setting up their tent within the past hour, he had again been confused and vomited before crawling into the tent and the warmth of his sleeping bag. It was shortly after he went into the tent that his body began to have a seizure. I can still remember the looks on his friends' faces. All were unshaven, haggard, faces drawn, skin reddened and leathery from the intense sun and wind, creases crisscrossed their faces from squinting into the sun, but most noticeable were their eyes. There was fear in their eyes, and I have seen this fear before. It was a fear of the unknown, a fear of death. At that point I had been a registered nurse for 27 years and had spent 2 years pre-hospital as an ambulance attendant, 10 years as an emergency room nurse in a Level 1 trauma center, and 10 years as an operating room nurse in a Level 1 trauma center. Throughout that time, I had seen more than my share of death and dying. I had seen that look of fear in my patients who were dying, and I have seen that same look on the faces of family members. It's distressful and despairing because the look is from deep within their souls and is looking for answers and hope.

I knew the despair, but what hope did this climber have? We were on a glacier at 7100 feet, surrounded by snow and tall mountains. The closest town, Talkeetna, was many miles away, and there were only two ways out, fly or hike. The flight would take 35 minutes, and the hike would take days to weeks because many rivers and lakes separated the two. To make matters worse, the weather had taken a drastic change: the clouds had dropped, and we were now "socked in," with no opportunity for rescue by plane or helicopter.

MyEverest Quote

"The time is always right to do what is right."
—Martin Luther King, Jr.

Being Open to Challenge

Before I did anything, I had to assess my situation to find out what medical supplies I had, what my resources were, and just how critical my patient was. The national park ranger provided me with a medical kit that contained a wide variety of drugs, syringes, intravenous solutions and tubing, bandages, splints, ointments, sutures, instruments, and almost everything that a medical person would need. What I was hoping to find was there, and it was plentiful. Dexamethasone was the drug of choice to reduce cerebral edema and given intravenously can create drastic changes. There were also intravenous solutions, but they were all cold and I could not start an intravenous infusion with cold fluids because I could potentially send this climber into shock, something that he did not need to add to his already grave situation. I asked the ranger to warm the fluids by putting the intravenous bag inside his parka and against his skin. This would take awhile! As far as resources, the national park ranger said he had medical training and experience to care for people with cuts, fractures, and headaches, but this was a little more complicated. I recalled that the climber's friends had mentioned that a doctor had given them advice at high camp, so I challenged the camp ranger to try to contact him by walkie-talkie.

Next, it was time to do a more thorough evaluation of the climber. I began my exam with a quick head-to-toe evaluation that I had adopted as an emergency room nurse. First, I noted his ABCs (airway, breathing, and circulation). I quickly observed that he was breathing, though labored, and with my hand on his wrist I felt a strong, bounding pulse. Then it was time to check for level of consciousness. The patient did not respond to the painful stimuli of me rubbing my knuckles on his chest. This is one way that we, as nurses, try to assess a patient's level of consciousness. Inflicting a stimulus of pain should elicit some type of response. As best as I could tell, his pupils were constricted and nonreactive to light. Examination of the pupils with a bright light can help identify cerebral issues. When listing pupil reaction, we normally note pupil size in millimeters, whether they are constricted or dilated, and how they respond to bright light. In a further exam of his breathing, I noted that his breaths were deep and labored and he had a large amount of sputum o,n his lips. It was not frothy, so I relaxed somewhat. Frothy sputum accompanied by labored breathing and chest pain at high altitudes could be symptoms of HAPE. In HAPE, there is poor air exchange in the lungs due to the altitude change; this results in a life-threatening form of pulmonary edema. Symptoms of this disease are fatigue, shortness of breath, crackling sounds in the chest, frothy pink sputum, and bluish lips. I found a stethoscope in the medical kit and used it to listen to his chest. I was relieved to hear good air exchange in the lower bases of the lungs.

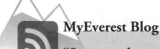

MyEverest Blog

"Some say that extreme adventure is too dangerous, that you might not live. But for the extremist, not to adventure is not to live."
—MC

As I continued my exam, I noted that his pants were soiled with urine. During a seizure patients can lose control of their bladder. Next, I turned to his friends to see whether they could give me any more health data on our patient, who continued to have seizures. Did they know anything about his medical history? Was he on any medications? Did he consume alcohol? Was he diabetic? All these questions and more I fired at his friends. I was now in my diagnostics mode and trying to do the best that I could on a glacier in the middle of the mountains. Only blank stares were returned because his friends knew nothing personal about this climber. Undaunted, I continued my assessment and applied a pulse oximeter (an LED unit that also measured pulse rate), which I also found in the medical kit. Pulse oximetry, a method of gauging the oxygen concentration of red blood cells as they circulate through the body, is achieved by applying a small probe on the end of a fingertip. These clothespin-like external probes are used on almost every mountain climb because the readings can aid in knowing whether or not a climber is having challenges associated with oxygenation. There are many reservations, though, when using these probes because altitude can greatly affect the readings, as can the sensitivity of the probe because cold digits may not produce a very desirable reading. In cold weather, the body shunts blood away from the extremities to the main organs as a method of self-preservation, so it would be expected for climbers to have cool-to-cold fingers, which are not conducive to accurate readings. To alleviate this situation, we climbers will normally warm our hands for some time so we can get a better reading. A normal reading would be 98–100% at sea level. After warming my patient's fingers for some time by wrapping them in my hand, I applied the probe and waited anxiously. Oximetry reading of 70%, and pulse rate of 100. At sea level, he would be close to death with this oxygen concentration level, but I had no benchmarks to compare it to at our altitude.

Believing in Self

However, one thing I knew was that it was not good. I asked the park ranger if he had an oxygen tank and tubing, and within minutes he was back in the tent with the requested supplies. I turned the tank on by twisting the dial on top and was relieved to see that the gauge registered "full." I connected one end of the oxygen tubing to the tank and the other end (the nasal cannula) to my patient by inserting the nasal prongs into his nares (nostrils). I adjusted the flow to 3 liters because I felt that was a negligible amount to help him become better oxygenated. I next checked his blood pressure with a sphygmomanometer and found it to be low: 96/60. He had been vomiting and was probably very dehydrated. He needed fluids, but they were still too cold! In the medical kit I found glucose paste and decided to rule out hypoglycemia. If he was diabetic and his blood sugar was dangerously low, this would help raise his level of consciousness. I applied the paste under his tongue (sublingual), hoping that absorption would be rapid. I was hoping against all hope that he would suddenly open his eyes, and all would be well. But it was not to happen. There were no noticeable changes.

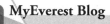

MyEverest Blog

You are one tough nurse and you have shown the world that not only can you live your dreams but you can do almost anything you set your mind to. Well done on completing your 7 summits project!—MC

It was right about this time, as I had finished my assessment, that the ranger stuck his head in the tent to tell me that he was in contact by walkie-talkie with the doctor higher up on the mountain. The connection was weak, and when he stepped inside the tent he lost the transmission. With experimentation we found that if he stood a short distance away from the tent, he could receive the doctor's transmissions. However, due to that distance away from the tent, we had to assemble a team to relay the message. Our transmission team consisted of the national park ranger receiving the message about 25 feet from the tent, who then conveyed it to one of the climber's friends halfway to the tent by yelling the message, who then conveyed the message to another friend just outside the tent, who then conveyed the message to me at the patient's side. It was trial and error in the beginning and very frustrating as I tried to relay vital signs and patient conditions to the doctor, while he tried to ask me more and more questions to get a better picture of what was really happening 10,000 feet below him. After a few minutes of too many people trying to speak in medicalese, a language unfamiliar to them for the most part, we transitioned to writing short notes that could easily be read and interpreted:

Doctor: What is his condition?
Nurse: Bad. BP 96/60, P 120, R 12, Pulse Ox 70%. Seizuring, nonresponsive to pain, PEARL at 2 mm.
Doctor: Have you given any medications?

Nurse: Yes. Glucose paste sublingual and O_2 at 4 litres.
Doctor: Do you have dexamethasone?
Nurse: Yes.
Doctor: Give 10 mg IV.
Nurse: IV fluids cold/IM?
Doctor: Give 8 mg IM now and 10 mg IV when fluids warm.
Nurse: OK.
Doctor: Do you have a Foley catheter?
Nurse: Yes.
Doctor: Insert Foley.

A Foley catheter is a sterile tube inserted into the bladder through the urethra to facilitate drainage of urine. It was right at this time that my guide stuck his head in the tent to announce that it was time to leave. The team was ready to head up the mountain, and they could not wait any longer. Before I could utter a word of protest, the park ranger spoke up as he, too, had entered the tent and said, "There is no damn way that this guy is leaving as he is the only thing that this patient has to prevent him from dying. And besides, I am the law on the mountain so I say he stays." I could see the fear in the ranger's eyes, but I also could see that he was in control, and even though this situation was way outside his comfort zone he still had confidence in what he saw was happening with my patient. My guide knew better than to complain as he, too, had seen death on the mountain and up until that moment had not known the severity of the situation. My presence and priority to do what matters most at that moment was the balance that was needed in this situation. I was here for a reason, one that was much more important than the summit of the mountain.

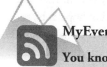

MyEverest Blog

You know that—after all, nurses are the best, but stubborn.—AC

Engaging in Risky Business

As we continued our treatment of the patient, my mind wandered, and I felt like I was back in the emergency room in Corpus Christi, Texas. In my mind, my best friend, Dr. David Gray, was giving me these orders as we smoothly and efficiently took care of the patient's needs as best we could. I was not alarmed and was very relaxed, because I had gone through this same algorithm of treatment regimens many times before. The climber's friends watching this event unfold could not see the fear in my eyes because

I had learned long ago to repress this feeling. My expression was cold, my movements methodical, and my actions well thought out. The doctor and I were a team, separated by 10,000 feet of ice, snow, and subzero temperatures. As I completed the catheterization of my patient, the ranger suddenly appeared to announce that the intravenous fluids that he had kept close to his chest were now warmed and at body temperature. Perfect timing. I cleaned up my supplies from the catheterization and inserted an intravenous needle into the patient's arm. After the tubing was connected, I opened the fluids to make certain that I had a patent connection. Then I reinforced the puncture site with adhesive and splints because I did not want the involuntary action of seizure activity to dislodge the catheter in the vein. Once secured, I administered a dose of dexamethasone, as ordered previously, and relayed a note back to the doctor that the Foley was in, intravenous started, and medications were given intravenously.

Unfortunately, the message was not delivered: the batteries had died in the walkie-talkie, and a frantic search had ensued in camp for replacements. Cold temperatures sap the energy out of batteries at a drastic rate, and normally they are kept by climbers close to their skin, or deep inside garments away from the cold. Minutes passed, and no change was noted so I administered a second dose. Now I was relying on my memory to guide me through administration of this medication. Within minutes of the second dose, my patient abruptly opened his eyes, looked up at me, and said, "Who the hell are you?" Sweeter words I have never heard because I had prepared myself for the worst-case scenario but was now pleasantly surprised to have my patient wake from a semi-comatose state. At the moment of his awakening I had been hovering above him, adjusting fluids, probes, and catheters, so I was unsure if he awoke from a dream or a nightmare, but nonetheless he awoke! "Quick, get his friends in here!" I yelled through the permeable tent walls. I needed my patient to see someone of whom he was familiar. A friend appeared in the tent and excitedly started to make conversation, and my patient responded appropriately. The friend's eyes, which had shown fear, were now full of hope as he tried to tell his incapacitated friend how worried they had been. My patient relayed to his friend that he had little recall of his summit bid, and no recall of the trip to Base Camp. He did remember experiencing the worst headache of his life and said that he felt like his head was going to explode. That feeling was gone now, but he was still sick.

MyEverest Quote

"Here I am safely returned over those peaks from a journey far more beautiful and strange than anything I had hoped for or imagined—how is it that this safe return brings such regret?"
—Peter Matthiessen

We arranged to move him to the national park ranger's tent, where there was more room and heat from a solar-powered generator. By this time the entire camp had heard of the perilous situation, and as we exited the climber's tent we were greeted with thunderous applause and all kinds of lifting help to move our patient from tent to tent. Then, using the camp ranger's walkie-talkie, which was alive again due to new batteries, I was able to personally give my faceless doctor a final report on our patient. I thanked him for his assistance, which was greatly appreciated, and he did likewise. We ended our conversation with his off-the-cuff remark about sending a bill for services rendered. That is one bill that won't be paid!

Dreaming the Impossible Dream

After my patient was secured in the park ranger's tent and resting comfortably, I discovered that the two of us were alone. I took advantage of this opportunity to talk with this man I had been treating for the past four hours. During treatment, I had many mental conversations with myself and wanted to share with him now what an ordeal this had been and how lucky he was to be alive. However, as anticlimactic as it could have been, my patient relayed to me that he had suffered from HACE on a previous climb and had been warned by his doctor to stay away from higher altitudes because he had had a near-death experience that time also! He lamented that he loved the mountains and needed to be there because it was "his fix" to keep him sane. My initial hurt and anger at his lack of reasoning, which could have caused other deaths besides his own, turned to understanding as I, too, had this need for the mountains and challenge. It's hard to understand the mind-set of a climber who knowingly will climb to higher altitude hoping against all odds that a previous affliction with HACE will not come back to haunt him on subsequent climbs. But then again, it is not very different from a race car driver injured in an accident who can't wait to drive again, or a pilot involved in a crash who wants to fly again. In the medical setting we see it as comparable to the cardiac patient who can't wait to be discharged from the hospital so that he can smoke, even though he knows it is killing him. Either way, the drive is strong and in both cases self-destructive.

I left my patient sitting up in the camp ranger's tent and wondered, as I walked away, if I had really saved his life, or if I had simply delayed the inevitable because by all accounts it sounded like he was going to continue mountain climbing. All I knew was that I had done as best I could with the resources at hand and knew for sure that I would not ever want to be on a future climbing team with him because he was a walking time-bomb, ready to explode and possibly incur collateral damage.

Rescues occur on the mountains often, and it was on **Mt. Everest** in 2006 that Dan Mazur, a well-known mountaineer and guide, saved Lincoln Hall's life near the summit of **Mt. Everest**. This rescue caused Dan to abort his—and his team's—bid for the summit. Dan's selflessness has been immortalized in this song:

DON'T WALK ON BY

Lyrics and melody by Mary Clare Reinhardt
Dedicated to Dan Mazur

Verse 1

> *When my brother takes a fall, am I there to lend a hand?*
> *Or do I walk on by. Um umm, um um um umm.*
> *Will I shut my open eyes? Will I cover up my ears?*
> *So I won't hear him cry. Um umm, um um um umm.*

Chorus

> *Don't walk on by, your fellow man.*
> *He's reaching out, to grasp your hand.*
> *You want your dream, it's just in sight.*
> *But in the end, just do what's right.*
> *Don't walk on by.*

Verse 2

> *Now I see it everywhere, it's the drive to get ahead.*
> *To make it to the top. Um umm, um um um umm.*
> *And the people walking by, with their heads up in the clouds.*
> *Do you think they'll stop? Um umm, um um um umm.*

Verse 3

> *When I finally reach the top, will I hold my head up high?*
> *And stand against the sky. Um umm, um um um umm.*
> *Like the heroes of the past, the great men from days gone by.*
> *That spirit will not die. Um umm, um um um umm.*

Finding the Balance

When I speak to my nursing students about balance in life, I use the analogy of juggling, with the balls representing responsibilities, priorities, things to do, places to go, and so on. As we know, the object is to keep all of those balls in the air without any of them hitting each other and/or striking the ground. When there are more balls in play, there is a greater challenge to keep all in the air, and at times occasional balls may be retrieved as they almost hit the ground. Controlling our spheres of activities is always a challenge, but we need to strive for that balance. To do so, it may require that we give up some of our activities because trying to do too much can result in a less than optimal performance. As nurses we are great jugglers; however, we always seem to have way too many balls in the air at any given time. Our challenge is to try to give up some of those balls of responsibility so that we are in control of our lives and have balance. We can have control over that balance, but in order to do so, we must assess our current condition. The best way to do that is to put pen to paper and try to figure out how balanced, or unbalanced, we really are as indicated by our activities. I've included Table 2-1 to help you get started.

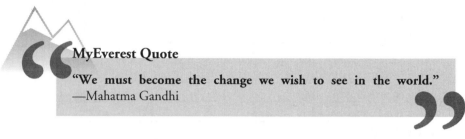

MyEverest Quote

"We must become the change we wish to see in the world."
—Mahatma Gandhi

Table 2–1 Balance Checklist

Review the following list to see how balanced you are in life.

Participation	Yes	No
Health		
• Participate in physical fitness regimen		
• Am member of sports team(s)		
• Eat a healthy diet		
• Sleep at least 8 hours		
• Get regular medical checkups		
• Get regular dental checkups		
• Need help		
Social		
• Am member of church or other religious group		
• Am member of religious committee(s)		
• Am member of community organization(s)		
• Am member of professional organization(s)		
• See movies often		
• Take vacations regularly		
• Visit family		
• Have a solid support system of family and friends		
• Shuttle kids to events		
• Speak to close friends often		
• Go out to dinner occasionally		
• Engage in laughter daily		
• Feel stressed out		
• Need help		

Participation	Yes	No
Work		
• Am employed full time		
• Am employed part time		
• Bring work home		
• Work overtime		
• Work on my day off		
• Work at more than one job		
• Enjoy my job		
• Say no when asked to do more work		
• Am stressed out		
• Need help		
School		
• Am enrolled in school full time		
• Am enrolled in school part time		
• Owe money on school loans		
• Am stressed out		
• Need help		

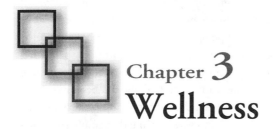

Chapter 3
Wellness

If I had my life to live over,
I'd try to make more mistakes next time.
I would relax. I would limber up.
I would be sillier than I have been.
I know of few things I would take seriously.
I would be crazier. I would be less hygienic.
I would take more chances.
I would take more trips.
I would climb more mountains, swim more rivers and watch more sunsets.
I would eat more ice cream and fewer beans.
I would have more actual problems and fewer imaginary ones.
I would not live prophylactically and sensibly,
and sanely hour after hour, day after day.
I have had my moments, and if I had to do it over again,
I'd have more of them, in fact I'd have nothing else.
Just moments, one after another, instead of living so many years
ahead of each day.
I would go places and do things and travel lighter than I have.
I would start barefoot earlier in the Spring and stay that way later in the Fall.
I would succeed by accident.
I would ride on more merry-go-rounds.
I would pick more daisies.
Worry is a cycle of inefficient thought ... whirling around a center of fear.
—BROTHER HERMAN E. ZACCARELLI

What is wellness in life, and who or what determines wellness? Just as balance in life is many things to many people, I believe that wellness in life is similar in that we have many ways to determine wellness and just as many ways to measure its value. Physical wellness, mental wellness, and financial wellness are but a few of the ways we can gauge our condition. I realize that from the medical perspective, wellness can be interpreted as reducing your risk for chronic disease, preventing and treating injuries, banishing environmental and safety hazards from your home and workplace, and eliminating unnecessary trips to the doctor, while at the same time making the best use of the healthcare system when you need it. However, I believe that wellness means much more than the absence of sickness and feel that it is a way of living that emphasizes such preventative measures as eating healthful foods, making exercise an enjoyable part of your life, and making self-care decisions that will actively improve the quality of your life. Many people feel that they have no control of their lives because they are over-whelmed with too many stimuli. The key to taking control is to focus on those things that we do control, and in doing so we start to control our life, rather than letting life lead us. Wellness is a daily event that begins when we eat a healthy breakfast and ends when we get a good night's sleep.

My Travels Through Life

Wellness in life always seemed to be a priority when growing up on the farm in rural Canada. Mom and Dad did the best that they could to provide for their litter of eight boys and one girl, yet it was always a challenge. Maintaining the physical, mental, and financial wellness of a large family was made that much more difficult by financial distress; Dad had to work two jobs just to make ends meet. I can remember that we were very well fed because we grew our own crops; raised and slaughtered our own poultry, beef, and pigs; and never lacked food. Our fitness regimen was balanced by active participation in sports at school, as well as the obligatory labor of strenuous farmwork, year round. With acreage to tend, animals to feed, and harvest to reap, we could never travel far from the farm for fear of neglecting our duties. At a very early age, I learned the valuable lessons of farm life, which I did not appreciate until much later.

Great Expectations

Contributing to these valuable lessons was the role model that my dad provided because he worked not only on our farm, but also as a city bus driver. The work required on the 100-acre farm challenged my dad, and he committed long hours to both jobs and had a lot of driving to do in between! His farm job went from 5:00 AM to 3:00 PM each day and after a 30-mile drive to the city, his job as a bus driver lasted from 4:00 PM to 12:30 AM. As kids growing up, we did not realize the sacrifices that he made for us. His primary goal was to keep us fed, clothed, and educated. Dad's education was completed in primary school because it was expected that he work on the family farm, which was the tradition in those days. He was adamant that none of us would be restricted in our pursuit of higher education because he realized early in life that his lack of schooling greatly limited his opportunities.

As was with any large farm family, one of our main purposes in life was to contribute to the betterment of the family by helping with the chores. Every day the animals had to be fed, milked, and cared for to various degrees. We could not get up and go to school without first spending an hour in the barn, day in and day out. It was required and had to be done. The only downside, besides getting up so early every day, was that we had no showers. Each day we went to school I am certain that some of the barn aroma was emitted from our clothes and body in a similar fashion to the cloud of dirt and dust that preludes Pigpen of Charlie Brown fame. Our school friends could always smell us coming—and let us know in no uncertain terms.

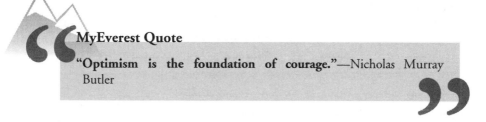

MyEverest Quote

"Optimism is the foundation of courage."—Nicholas Murray Butler

Another challenge was our family's limited financial status. As the family grew, so did our bodies, and clothes were an expensive commodity. The lone taxi driver in my hometown of Almonte, Ontario, took us to heart and on a monthly basis would drop off used clothes. His visits were Christmas-like because each article of clothing was like a present from God. We were eternally appreciative. However, I can recall on more than a few occasions when a fellow classmate would ridicule me for wearing a particular type of clothing that had been donated to the local Catholic Church for the needy by that same student's family. It was embarrassing, but we had little money to purchase new clothes. I can recall getting a pair of gloves for Christmas that were mismatched, only to find out later that Dad had retrieved them from the lost-and-found bin where he worked on the bus in the city. At least they kept my hands warm.

The Power of Family

Helping me overcome the challenge of dealing with patients suffering from emotional and psychiatric disorders were lessons learned from my only sister, Mary Ann. My sister Mary Ann was born with Down syndrome but died from non-Hodgkin's lymphoma at age 18. Mary Ann was an oasis in a sea of brothers, and she was surrounded by eight of the most loving brothers that any sister could ever have. I will always re-member Mary Ann as an angel who came into our lives. She brightened our days with her childish play and naivety, and her smile and soft voice made her a child forever. It was through her experiences in the school system that I came to understand the issues that existed for mentally challenged children, and it was those challenges that led me to realize that Mary Ann had given me a gift that I never had anticipated. When Mary Ann transitioned from a special school for challenged kids to the mainstream schools, she would bring her friends home with her to play. It was through those kids that I learned of the taunting and ridicule that the "normal" kids would bestow upon them. The gift that I acquired from my sister was the ability to interact very comfortably with mentally challenged kids and to advocate for them on every level. I will always have an affinity in my heart for the less fortunate and downtrodden and have Mary Ann to thank for making me a better person.

MyEverest Blog

Happy Nurses Week. "Unless we are making progress in our nurs-ing every year, every month, every week—take my word for it we are going back." Florence Nightingale, 1914.—SD

Prescription for Health

As nurses, we are taught that there are three stages of illness prevention: primary, secondary, and tertiary. We are taught that there were many things we could do to prevent a disease from either occurring, progressing, or, after a person had acquired a disease, becoming worse. These lessons came in quite handy as Carol and I traveled often, and in most cases, were exposed to a wide array of diseases. It was December 1988, and 5 months had passed since we left our home in Corpus Christi, Texas. We were backpacking around the world for an entire year and had just spent Christmas in the apartment of a fellow traveler who lived in Hong Kong. It was time for our booster shots of gamma globulin, to prevent hepatitis A, which was available in a local pharmacy without a prescription.

Needles and medications in hand, as well as Christmas cards from family and friends, we walked back to our apartment to get ready for our trip into China the next day. Once settled in, with bags packed, letters read, and time for sleep, I drew the medication up into separate syringes, 3 cc each. I gave Carol her injection, as I had given thousands, with light hand and little complaint. However, now it was her turn. In training to become a certified public accountant (CPA), she admittedly noted that she missed the class on how to give injections. With a few minutes of instruction, and a lot of reassurance, Carol plunged the needle deep into my hip. After she injected the medication, hands trembling and voice quivering, she quickly withdrew the needle, asking if all had gone well. I joked that the injection was the worst I had ever received, and then asked if she had withdrawn the barrel of the syringe prior to injecting the medicine, to make certain that she had not injected the contents into a major blood vessel. I have never seen Carol look as shell-shocked. She was slow to admit that she had forgotten to do so as directed and asked what could have happened if the medication had gone into the bloodstream. Again, I joked that I could possibly stop breathing and die within the next 8 hours as a result of this potential mistake. I thought nothing more of it as we immediately went to sleep in preparation for a big day of travel.

It was early the next morning when I awoke to see Carol lying beside me, wide awake, with a look of concern on her face, that I sensed a problem. I asked what was up, and Carol responded that she had lay awake all night listening to me breathing, ready to give me mouth-to-mouth respirations, should I stop breathing. I looked at her quizzically and wondered why she was saying this, but then remembered our medication injections and late-night conversation regarding potential mistakes. I smiled out of love and then cowered out of fear of retaliation as I told Carol my flippant remark was just that: a joke. I did not contract hepatitis during that trip but suffered her wrath because she would not let me forget the cruel joke I had played on her that night.

My Journey in Nursing

In the first class of the semester, I always ask my students why they have chosen to pursue a degree in nursing. Over the years, I have been surprised by a number of their answers. Most students have sought guidance and been given direction before choosing this path, while others simply made a last minute decision with no thought given to the enormity of the challenge that lies ahead.

Life-Changing Decisions

As a student nurse, there were many occasions when wellness, both mental and social, became problematic as I struggled to graduate from school. Early in my student life those challenges surfaced when I had to begin assuming the responsibility of caring for the various needs of my patients. Prior to entering school to become a nurse, I had never set foot in a hospital, so I had no idea what to expect when dealing with people who were sick and dying. My first summer job during nursing school was in a psychiatric hospital, where I really got to do a lot of bedside nursing. It was here that I saw my first patient having a seizure and was dumbstruck by the involuntary motions that I had read about in school. Later the next day I was also able to attend the autopsy of this same patient, which confirmed for me that I was able to tolerate the worst that nursing had to throw at me. However, little did I know then that it would get much worse!

During my second summer of school, I worked as an ambulance attendant, and it was during this job that I began to see a side of human tragedy that I had never imagined. I will never forget my very first ambulance call; it was a multi-car accident on a freeway late at night. At the scene I had to look for people who had been ejected from one of the cars into the bush along the side of the road. I will never forget the mutilated, lifeless bodies. This was just the beginning of a future career as an ambulance attendant and an inkling of what lay ahead in my career as a nurse.

As nurses, we learned that wellness means reducing your risk for chronic disease, preventing and treating injuries, and eliminating unnecessary trips to the doctor—all while making the best use of the healthcare system when you need it. As nurses we care for the sick and help them to regain their health and wellness. This restoration of health occurs through our care while the patient is hospitalized and through our lessons of how to care for themselves after their discharge. However, I have always maintained that in order to effectively care for our patients, we first need to take better care of ourselves. Unfortunately, though, this is an area in which I believe we fail ourselves, and subsequently our patients.

As patient advocates, we always put the patients' needs first because this is what we have learned in school; however, in doing so, we sometimes set ourselves up to fail. We often neglect our own health and welfare as a result: more often than not, we as nurses have to deal with our own medical conditions induced from attentiveness to our patients, rather than ourselves. Many colleagues over the years have attributed chronic bladder problems, whether right or wrong, to the fact that they have not gone to the bathroom when they felt the urge because they were too busy with their patients. And many more have blamed weight gain on lack of time to eat; they religiously devour fast foods and snacks in their haste to get back to their patients. And then there are those who have allowed themselves to fall out of shape as the hectic pace, long shifts, and increasing demands of patient care have dominated their lives to the point that they live only for work and their family, with little attention to themselves.

MyEverest Blog

Awesome! Nice Job! Sweet As! Thank God! Whew! Boy Oh Boy! At Last! Oh Man! Fantastic! Congratulations! Good Work! You Beauty! What else can I say?—MC

What Kind of Person Do You Want to Be?

The adage that we nurses are our own worst patients resonates truth because if we can't effectively take care of ourselves, how can we begin to take care of our patients? I like to use the analogy of the message delivered by airline attendants as they address safety prior to takeoff. We can probably all recite this message, especially if you fly often: "If you have someone that needs assistance with application of the oxygen mask … put yours on first and then help them with their mask!" The message is that we have to take care of ourselves before we can take care of others! As nurses we do a *great* job of advocating for our patients (which is admirable), but in doing so we neglect ourselves! So, how do we develop our wellness? Well, it's as simple as establishing a fitness routine accompanied by proper nutrition and a good night's sleep.

> ## MyEverest Quote
>
> **"Strength does not come from physical capacity. It comes from an indomitable will."**—Mahatma Gandhi

In 1998, I developed a presentation for my perioperative colleagues titled "PMS (Physical, Mental, Stress) Relief in the Operating Room," and it was intended to address my concerns related to the physical, mental, and social health of my fellow nurses. As a former member of the National Board of Directors for the Association of periOperative Registered Nurses (AORN), I was able to present this information to my colleagues as I traveled around the country doing presentations on leadership. As a perioperative nurse, I knew the stressors of the work environment and had seen way too many of my friends developing chronic illnesses that they said were related to the work environment, but I believe were due to their lack of ability to deal with the stressors in that environment. When physically healthy, we nurses are better able to carry out our everyday tasks without being overly tired; when mentally healthy, we like ourselves for our achievements, learn from our mistakes, and are able to adjust to life's demands; and when in healthy social relationships, we are able to get along with others, have friends, respect the rights of others, know how to give, and, most importantly, accept help.

To Risk or Not to Risk

However, to achieve this state of wellness, I inferred that nurses must first know, choose, and then practice those behaviors that promote wellness. The biggest challenge, though, was distinguishing the risk behaviors that lead away from wellness and healthy behaviors such as making the time to work out, knowledge of proper nutrition, ergonomics in the work setting, and competing claims such as family, kids, and personal commitments. I addressed those barriers to wellness in my presentations because to overcome these barriers is to start on the path to wellness.

MyEverest Blog

You guys obviously worked so hard for this well deserved summit of the highest mountain in the world. So proud of you guys!!! You are tough, courageous, diligent, and come prepared. What I love the most is that you all had a dream and you pursued it. Fantastic! You are all inspirations!—MC

To address physical health I recommended adopting a physical fitness regimen that started with a basic walking program and included taking the stairs instead of elevators. In addition, I advocated for well-balanced meals because the standard "nurse's breakfast" of coffee, coffee, and more coffee, accompanied by snacks for lunch, does not set us up well to make it through our long shifts. When addressing mental health, I discussed body image and our dissatisfaction with self both physically and as a person. The average American woman is 5'3" and weighs 150 pounds; yet with role models in the media portrayed as gaunt thin, it is easy to imagine the challenges that nurses have in trying to identify healthy body image. And finally, when addressing social health, I explored the challenges that exist when trying to maintain healthy relationships both in our personal lives with our families and loved ones and in the work environment with our colleagues on the healthcare team. I completed my presentation by challenging nurses to determine where they are in regard to wellness, to take measures to overcome those barriers that exist from establishing overall wellness, to become more aware of stressors both at home and work, and, most importantly, to develop strategies to deal with those stressors.

MyEverest Blog

You have touched many of us and honestly have all of perioperative nursing (as well as many more) waiting to have you tell your story.—PG

Weathering the Storm

As on the mountains, there are storms in our healthcare environments. And, as on the mountains, the storms in health care are related to our ever-changing climate. Change is a constant in health care, and with change there is stress. The stressors in nursing are many and include changes in technology, hectic pace, lack of staff, doing more with less, reimbursement, and patient-safety incidents. Stress is a natural reaction to everyday challenges and changes, and what's most important is not the stress itself, but how we react to it. To achieve our maximum potential as nurses, we must have better control of stress management, which includes an awareness of the physical effects of stress and the ability to minimize those effects. Our ability to cope with those stressors is what makes the difference in our ability to function as nurses in the healthcare environment. The most prevalent stressor in health care seems to be conflict in the workplace, which is a daily occurrence due to lateral violence from nurses, challenges from physicians, and anxiety on behalf of patients and families. Communications among all of these groups is the basis of our existence, yet seems most problematic because many people are challenged by less than effective communication skills. This is evidenced by The Joint Commission data that reflect communication as the number one reason in healthcare settings for sentinel events. Effective communication is a vital aspect of patient care, and teamwork and should be a priority in all situations, as it is on the mountain.

So, how do we deal with these constant stressors in the workplace and school environment? In keeping with my theme of the 7 Summits of Life, I recommend these 7 steps to a stress-free life:

1. Do a needs assessment of the stresses in your life; then make a list of those stressors as well as a list of potential strategies for stress reduction.
2. Prioritize the needs on your list, and develop those resources because you need to start now.
3. While you're starting to work on that list, smile often: this will not only make you feel better, but will also send a message to others that you are happy.
4. Follow that smile with daily laughter; this has been proven to lower blood pressure and reduce tension.
5. While you are smiling and laughing, try listening to your favorite music; it has been proven to reduce heart rate and blood pressure.
6. When starting to feel stressed, try to control your breathing; short and shallow breaths can lead to increased heart rate and feelings of tension and anxiety.
7. Start now with small steps toward wellness such as eating healthy meals, developing an exercise regimen, and doing something special for yourself.

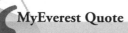

MyEverest Quote

"Pain is temporary. Quitting lasts forever."—Lance Armstrong

My Climbs on the Mountains

On the mountains, there were many occasions when overall wellness played a vital role in the success of the climb. In fact, it was on my first mountain of the 7 Summits, **Mt. Aconcagua** in Argentina, that the overall wellness of others became problematic for my own survival. January 12, 2001, started earlier for me than most days because it was simply an extension of the day before. The midnight hour passed, as did the hour previous, with nary a difference as life near the top of the continent of South America seemed frozen in time. And frozen it was: at 21,000 feet the tent that I was in was being torn off the mountain by violent winds, and the temperature had plummeted to –20 degrees Fahrenheit. My head was pounding with the increased altitude, and I knew that I had to drink more fluids to alleviate some of my symptoms. However, that meant getting completely dressed in down jacket and pants, applying crampons to boots, walking out into the cold to dig more snow to melt, and then melting and boiling the snow to make water. This had been the routine for the past 3 weeks; however, neither my tent-mate nor I had much energy left because the earlier push that day to high camp had exhausted us. Slowly, though, we did take turns working with our guides to keep an endless supply of snow ready for the stove. Preparation and practice makes us perfect, they told us; however, I felt that we had practiced enough.

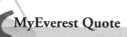

MyEverest Quote

"The race does not always go to the swift, but to those who keep on running."—Anonymous

The summit hour approached, and as professed, our preparation paid off. We left the tents with Nalgene bottles full of life-saving water, pockets crammed with hand warmers and power bars, and extra clothes jammed into our backpacks. The brutal winds added to the challenge of altitude as our team began our slow ascent to the summit. When our four-man team approached the canella, we discovered that two of our members had raised clear blebs on their faces, a direct result of the worsening cold magnified by the bone-chilling winds. Frostbite may be classified according to the depth of tissue injury. First-degree frostbite involves the superficial skin and is characterized by erythema and anesthesia. Clear blebs are associated with second-degree injury. In third-degree frostbite, hemorrhagic vesicles indicate deeper subcutaneous injury. Finally, injury to muscle and bone are seen with fourth-degree frostbite. It was clearly evident that these two teammates had second-degree frostbite and needed to

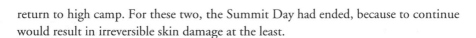

return to high camp. For these two, the Summit Day had ended, because to continue would result in irreversible skin damage at the least.

Importance of Your Beliefs

They say that misery loves company, and company we had, as other climbers from teams all over the world had joined us to share in the triumph of standing atop the highest mountain in South America. However, it seemed that many of these team members were not privy to the knowledge that preparation meant survival; to tempt fate in this hostile environment was tantamount to inviting disaster. As I continued straight up the narrow route, I began to encounter these ill-prepared climbers, and my heart went out to those who were immobile on the trail, freezing to death from lack of clothing, and dehydrated due to lack of water. The nurse in me took over the mountain climber who was struggling to survive, and I began to dispense water, food, hand warmers, and even extra clothes. How could I allow these people to die, even though they had set themselves up to fail? My guide was reluctant for me to stop and dispense these goods; he kept repeating that I had to take care of my self. Again, the curse of nursing … always feeling that we have to take care of others despite their inability to care for themselves. Even here at 21,000 feet, the cause-and-effect relationship still continues! I will always remember one climber, a young German woman, who was crying very loudly and saying that her feet were frozen and could not feel any sensation. Her guide stood by helplessly as I removed her boots, rubbed her feet vigorously, applied a heavier pair of my extra socks, and left a foot warmer pad in each boot. She was still crying when I left her, but I believe some of those tears were from her appreciation. Another climber required water, and yet another needed a power bar, and so it went as I continued my climb to the summit. With the summit in site, and the climb almost over, I started to feel the euphoria of the altitude, and I gave myself away to the giddiness of triumph as I stepped onto the roof of South America, at 23,000 feet.

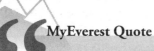

" MyEverest Quote

"The journey, not the arrival, matters."—T. S. Eliot **"**

The euphoria of the moment continued, but despite my triumphant summit I was having a hard time grasping the reality of the situation. For some reason, I had wanted to continue climbing upward, yet there was no place further to climb. Beneath my feet and inside my gaze were the majesty of the Andean peaks, all snow covered and triumphant in their own way, yet the view was starting to blur and the skies were a brilliant blue. My head was pounding again, but this time it felt like a vise had also been applied and was squeezing on my temples with painful force. After the obligatory photos, it was time to depart the summit, and we stopped briefly to refuel with power bars and fluids. The descent would be tedious, to say the least. It was then that I discovered that in my haste to help others on the climb to the summit I had shortchanged myself: I was now out of fuel, both literally and figuratively. I had no supplies left, and my body's gas tank was running on empty. My internal engine sputtered on the first step off the summit, and my body stalled. I could not put my feet firmly on the ledge where they should have been. I fell, sliding forward to the next ledge, where a well-placed boulder prevented my departure off the side of the mountain into the thin air of the Andes.

My guide appeared, quickly evaluated the situation, and determined that I would have to be "short-roped" down the mountain, which required that I be tethered to him by a short piece of rope. This insurance factor was needed because I had become dehydrated and weakened due to a lack of fuel for my body.

MyEverest Blog

I have been following you all the way up and down the mountain— holding my breath at times, and praying that you would be safe. Thanks so much for the detailed blogs that have allowed me to climb Everest from the comfort of my home.—PP

By helping others to succeed, I had inadvertently hurt myself. I cannot remember much of the descent but do recall quite a few falls that were controlled by the rope attached securely from my harness to my guide's harness. My wife Carol vividly recalls my satellite phone call a few days off the summit and felt certain that I would never climb again because my weakened state caused her so much alarm. I do remember feeling like my body had endured a heavyweight boxing match, but was I the winner or the loser? I had learned a valuable lesson on **Mt. Aconcagua**: that overall wellness is as important to the success of a climb as it is to patient care in the hospital; however, I had to be careful in extending myself to those who had not prepared as well as they should, because doing so limited my ability to help myself. This challenge would haunt me in future climbs, as well as in life, because more times than not I have continued to extend myself to others when they should have done more to prepare themselves.

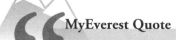

MyEverest Quote

"The wise man travels to discover himself."—James Russell Lowell

While climbing **Mt. McKinley**, Alaska, in December 2003, it was my overall state of physical wellness that turned one of my biggest physical challenges into a success because my preparations had prepared me for the ultimate climb in less than favorable conditions. Six months before this climb, I determined that I would need to train more because I felt that I would be challenged on the mountain, and true to form I was challenged as never before. My daily routine until that point had been to run for at least an hour, do an hour of sit-ups and push-ups, and do at least 6–8 flights of stairs 2–3 times. In my research, I found that in addition to carrying heavy loads in backpacks on **Mt. McKinley**, it was also required that climbers pull sleds packed with gear. In order to train for this obstacle, I acquired a child's wagon, loaded it with 100 pounds of weight, and devised a harness that connected me to the wagon. I then loaded my backpack with 75 pounds of weights and water bottles, connected myself to the wag-

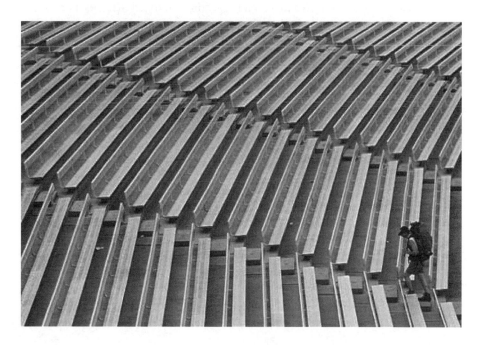

on, and proceeded to walk, pulling these weights along my running route, which now turned into a torturous route of pain and suffering. Kids and car drivers looked at me in amazement as I fought not only the weight of my loads, but the stifling summer heat of South Carolina. Temperatures of well over 100 degrees would be replaced 6 months later by temperatures that dropped to –50 degrees.

Being Proactive

This training would prove to be lifesaving on **Mt. McKinley**. Directly in front of me on the trail, just after breakfast, a fellow climber slipped into a crevasse after falling through a snow bridge and was supported in the crevasse only by his upper arms. It took four of us to pull him out because he was very tall and heavy. His worst injury seemed to be his back, which he had twisted and strained during the fall. He brushed off the fall and laughed about it, but I could see the pain on his face as he made his way back into the line directly in front of me. Due to the crevasses in this area, we were all roped together to avoid injury and fatal falls, and subsequently our pace was dictated by the person in front of us. After the fall the pace slowed noticeably: the climber who had fallen was having a hard time pulling his sled, and the grimaces on his face indicated that he was in pain. At a rest stop a few hours later, I asked if I could help, and he confided that he had just had back surgery prior to the trip and was now worried that he could not continue because his pain was extreme. He admitted that he had just taken two very strong narcotics but begged me not to tell the guide because he wanted to continue climbing as long as he could and was hopeful that the pain would stop. I offered to lighten his load and placed over half of his fuel tank supply on my sled, which greatly increased my load but was tolerable due to my extensive training.

MyEverest Blog

"The journey is the destination and the destination is the beginning of a new journey."—MC

For the rest of that day I was pushed to the limit of my fitness as I pulled a heavily weighted sled, but I did so to help a fellow climber. That night in camp I volunteered to examine him for further injuries, and after doing so I determined that he could not climb any farther. His pain radiated from his back to his toes, was made extremely worse by weight bearing, and he now was not able to carry any weight at all! An inability to bear weight was suicide on the mountain, and this climber was actually very fortunate that we were only 2 days from Base Camp. He bristled at the idea of having to leave the mountain; he had planned for years in advance to be here. But he realized that he could not move forward: his condition was made barely tolerable by the narcotics he self-administered. We all hated to see a team member having to leave prematurely but knew that it was best for him and for the team. Plans were made to take him back to Base Camp that next day: his sled would be emptied and used as a stretcher, which the guides would pull along the snow.

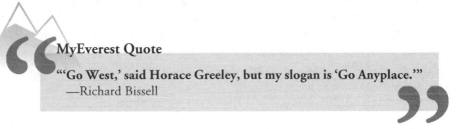

MyEverest Quote

"'Go West,' said Horace Greeley, but my slogan is 'Go Anyplace.'"
—Richard Bissell

Illness became an issue for me on **Mt. Elbrus** in Russia as a respiratory infection and high fever almost ended my summit bid. Prior to departure for Russia, I had been fighting off a cold and was taking many over-the-counter medications to coun-

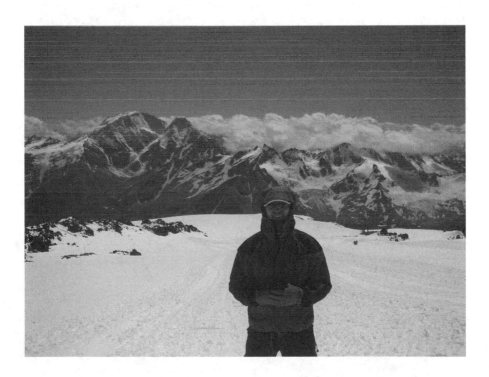

teract the symptoms of headache, stuffy nose, sore throat, and a productive cough. I noticed upon arrival in Moscow that I was very tired and lethargic but blamed it on the transatlantic flight and subsequent flights across Europe to my final destination. Within a few days of arrival in Russia, I was at Base Camp for our climb and had spared little time in worrying about my symptoms, which had gotten worse and now prevented me from sleep. Our campsite consisted of gigantic oil barrels that had been converted to sleeping quarters and gave rudimentary protection from the weather. This camp would double as both base and advance camp for the climbers, and, as would be our routine on most mountains, we arrived in camp that morning and planned to summit that next night. Due to a luggage issue, my medications did not accompany me to southern Russia, so I had to beg, borrow, and plead to get medicines to help alleviate my symptoms, the worst of which was now a fever that caused almost uncontrollable shaking.

Persist Until You Succeed

The midnight hour approached, and we geared up for our summit bid despite raging wind, blowing snow, and subzero temperatures. Headlamps in place, we traced our way across the barren snowscape; the snow now appeared to be blowing sideways. Our down clothing protected us from the cold, and our snow goggles prevented snow from blinding us as we trudged obediently through the night following our Russian guide. My chills continued throughout the climb—in the beginning I thought it was the cold winds finding their way through my clothes, but only later did I realize that it was the fever causing the shaking. As I neared the summit, the snow had increased and we were truly in a whiteout: we could not see much farther than a few feet in front of us when we stepped onto the top of Europe. I remember reaching that summit, sitting there to rest, and not wanting to get up again because I felt so exhausted.

> **MyEverest Quote**
>
> "Leave nothing for tomorrow which can be done today."
> —Abraham Lincoln

The climb itself had not been that tough, as compared to others, but I felt worse on the summit than I had on any other. Why was I so exhausted? Why was I so tired? I slowly left the summit and fell in pace behind my team, but after a short while I could barely see them in front of me. I finally caught up to them at a rest break, and it was here that the team questioned my energy level because on prior practice climbs I had done extremely well and was usually in the lead. One of the other climbers, an emergency medical technician (EMT), noted my lethargy and after a quick inspection commented that I was burning up with a fever. I had run out of Tylenol 12 hours earlier and had not hydrated as I should have so I felt worse than ever. A fellow climber offered to carry my pack, and our leader assigned one of the Russian guides to escort me to Base Camp. As the team departed, I got up to leave and noticed that my gait was imbalanced. Maybe it was the fact that I no longer was wearing my backpack, or maybe it was because I was extremely weak. As the sun rose, the snowstorm abated, and I now had to deal with the intensity of the morning heat. Putting one foot in front of the other became problematic, and we stopped to rest frequently. At each stop, my guide would pull out a cigarette, light it, and smoke the entire thing, while I sat across from him gasping for breath and burning up under the sun and from the fever that now had complete control of my body. With each stop came a new start as we would get up again to trudge through the snow ever so slowly. And with each start there was always a supportive glance from my guide to make certain that I was able to do what needed to be done. And so this routine was repeated as we played stop and go all the way down the mountain, although it never was a game.

> **MyEverest Quote**
>
> "**The greatest glory in living lies not in never falling, but in rising every time we fall.**"—Nelson Mandela

As we reached the edge of camp, members of my team came out to drag me the last few steps to the oil barrels. As much as I wanted them to carry me, because by now I was almost delirious with fever, my guide wanted me to walk those last few steps myself. To have them help me at the end would take away from this most difficult challenge that I had just completed! I made those last few steps and collapsed into my sleeping bag. Twelve hours later I awoke, just in time for our celebratory supper with our team. I entered the oil barrel that served as mess hall and was greeted with thunderous applause from my team. Initially they had not understood the reason for my lack of energy, but after conferring with the team guide they had found out how sick I had been and now were congratulating me for my efforts to climb despite my sickness.

Just prior to collapsing in my sleeping bag that morning my guide had found an American doctor in another climbing team, and he provided me with a Z-pak of antibiotics, Tylenol, energy drinks, and lots of fluids. By the time I walked into the mess hall, I was already on the mend and was able to enjoy the team celebration of our summit. It was a time to celebrate victories, and I wanted to share my appreciation with my guide who had escorted me down the mountain. Because he had guided me to our camp I gave him my very expensive headlamp as a token of appreciation, because it is used to guide us during the darkest hours. It seemed only fitting that he receive this present because it was during my darkest hours of ill health that he guided me back to life!

When we think of wellness, we need to think holistically and look at the entire picture: physical, mental, and financial. As I mentioned earlier in this chapter, on airline flights we are reminded of our need for wellness in the well-scripted safety message delivered by flight attendants. We are cautioned that if there is a need for oxygen, we should attach our own oxygen mask first before attempting to help others. The analogy holds true with nursing. If we are going to help our patients, we need to first take care of ourselves, otherwise we will not be helping them to attain the level of wellness that they so desperately need. Attaining a holistic level of wellness is challenging, to say the least, but with a structured plan, a support system, and a desire to better oneself it is well within our reach.

Table 3-1   Wellness Checklist

Review the following list to see how much wellness you have in life.

Wellness Activity	Yes	No
Physical		
• Had a complete health assessment (physical) in the last year		
• Have blood pressure checked at least once yearly		
• Had an eye examination in the last 3 years		
• Had a dental examination in the last 6 months		
• Don't smoke		
• Eat several servings of fruits and vegetables every day		
• Have eliminated fried foods from my diet		
• Sleep restfully 6 to 8 hours each night		

Wellness Activity	Yes	No
• Schedule intense cardio activity at least 5 days per week, 30 minutes per session, in addition to my activities of daily living		
Mental		
• Prioritize spending time with friends and loved ones		
• Spend time each day practicing stress management		
• Pray, reflect, and count blessings when starting the day and before going to bed		
• Read something inspirational or listen to good music		
• Have told somebody else I loved them or cared for them		
• Have a sense of belonging, meaning, and purpose in my life		
Financial		
• Have a stable job		
• Balance checkbook monthly		
• Pay off credit-card bill in full each month		
• Pay my bills immediately		
• Do not buy things to fill an emotional void		
• Am not in debt		

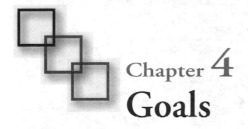

Chapter 4
Goals

People are often unreasonable, illogical, and self-centered;
Forgive them anyway.
If you are kind,
People may accuse you of selfish, ulterior motives;
Be kind anyway.
If you are successful, you will win some false friends
And some true enemies;
Succeed anyway.
If you are honest and frank, people may cheat you;
Be honest and frank anyway.
What you spend years building, someone could destroy overnight;
Build anyway.
If you find serenity and happiness, they may be jealous;
Be happy anyway.
The good you do today, people will often forget tomorrow;
Do good anyway.
Give the world the best you have, and it may never be enough;
Give the world the best you've got anyway.
You see, in the final analysis, it is between you and God;
It was never between you and them anyway.
—MOTHER TERESA

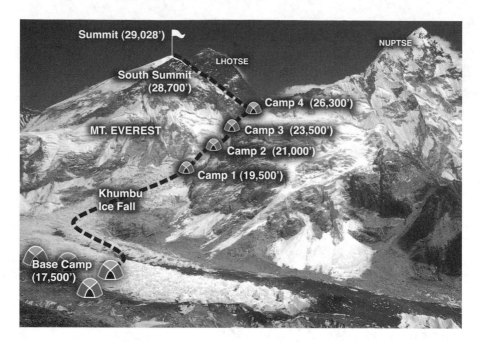

What are goals, and why do so many people say that they are important? Does everyone need them, and how do you get them? Is there a time frame for obtaining them, and, if so, at what age? According to Merriam-Webster's Collegiate Dictionary, 11th edition, a *goal* is an "end toward which effort is directed."

We all have Everests in our lives, such as professional goals, financial goals, health and wellness goals, or in my case even climbing **Mt. Everest** itself! Goals are the dreams that drive us to succeed and to seek our highest pursuits. However, all of those dreams and goals, those individual Everests, share one thing in common: the crevasses, obstacles, and challenges that prevent us from reaching our summits. What is your Everest? What crevasses stand between you and that summit? And what is the ladder that will get you across that crevasse and to the top?

When establishing goals, people often make the mistake of not setting dates or time frames, being too vague, and failing to write them down for future reference. Both personal and professional goals, as well as those of spouses, children, and other family members, if applicable, should be identified. Additionally, we should be able to distinguish between short-, mid-, and long-term goals, the influence of outside forces on those goals, and the obstacles that impede reaching those goals.

Ideally, we write these goals down, categorize them into the different areas of our life, such as education, career, travel, health, and so on, and then review the list frequently. Accomplished goals are deleted from the list, and new goals are added. I write mine on a legal pad that I call my "bucket list of things to do"; they are numbered, listed by date, and given a priority level. I leave room for additional information specific to obstacles along the way, and then take great satisfaction in drawing a line through the goal once completed. Goals motivate us to do better and once completed are achievements. By establishing goals, we are drawing a plan to help us to reach our potential.

MyEverest Blog

I never miss a day reading your blog and keeping up with your progress towards your goal. I plan to pledge a hundred dollars to the Summit Scholarship and I figure if 300 nurses total would do that then your initial goal would be reached. Keep on working towards the top of Mt. Everest and I know you will achieve that especially since you are so determined and always remembering safety comes first. I look forward to each day reading about your progress. Best wishes.—SD

My Travels Through Life

When I was a child, I never had goals, or never realized that I did, but I now know that Mom and Dad had developed some for me. My advancement through the Catholic primary school system was evidence of their establishment of educational goals for me, and I am forever in their debt for their vision because those primary school days shaped me into who I am today. My earliest recall of developing my own goals may have been in high school, when I decided to participate in competitive sports. Challenging me at that time, though, was my asthmatic condition, which was made worse by a decree handed down by our family doctor. His concern was valid: he warned that I should never run because it could initiate an asthma attack and probable hospitalization. Repeated asthma attacks as a young child usually followed playground activity at school and often necessitated trips to the local emergency room. Subconsciously, it may have been those early exposures to the medical setting that piqued my future interest in becoming a nurse. I see a similar sentiment in many of my students: early exposure to personal medical problems, or those of family members or friends, has been a pivotal reason for choosing nursing as a profession.

The Test for Success

However, despite the daily episodes of exercise-induced shortness of breath, the subsequent high-pitched sound of wheezing, and the lack of energy after an attack, I still wanted to participate on a team. As a youngster, I was shielded from farmwork by my Mom because hay fever, an allergy to animal hair, and my asthma crippled me to the point where I could not function. Airway-opening medical inhalers offered only temporary relief, and the attacks became more debilitating. Mom decided very early in my life that it would be easier for me to work in the house, rather than in the barn, so most of my chores were house-based. Of course I had exposure to all of the daily events of farm life and did my share of cutting, raking, and baling hay, as well as spreading manure, milking cows, and raising poultry. However, my exposures to the farmwork were limited and tempered by asthma attacks.

MyEverest Blog

You had a goal and you persevered and accomplished what you set out to do!!! You should be very proud!—KH

So, when I set the goal of becoming a member of a high school sports team it came as quite a shock to an overbearing mother who did not want to see her child suffer through more attacks of respiratory distress. Perhaps my goal was not realistic and not well thought out because my dream was to become a member of the football team. This rough-and-tumble sport, which demands a high level of physical fitness and conditioning, became my first conscious goal as I began to lay the foundation to become a successful athlete. Unknown to both my family doctor and my mom, I began to challenge myself to become an athlete by running home from school. The 3-mile trip started as a run/walk with frequent stops to catch my breath. However, eventually, with proper pacing and breathing control, I was able to do the entire distance without having to stop. This milestone in fitness gave meaning to my life because I had always been cautioned not to overexert myself for fear of respiratory complications. This accomplishment motivated me to continue my pursuit of a position on the football team. Months later, after a rigorous tryout and the biggest test to my respiratory system, I made the team. All of that running practice had paid off: my small size did not position me to be the best hitter or tackler, but throw me the ball, and I could run with it!

The Power of Goals

I have always felt that goal accomplishment should be celebrated, and not simply passed over, because more often than not, someone put a lot of pain and suffering into successful completion of that goal. It was 1983, and Carol and I were living in Corpus Christi, Texas. She had been very busy working full time and going to school full time

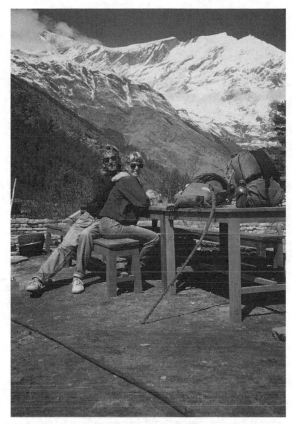

as she worked to complete her certified public accountant (CPA) program. I was busy working in the emergency room of a Level 1 trauma center and preparing to write my certification exam to become a certified emergency nurse (CEN). Both of us were burning the candle at both ends, so we took a night off to enjoy an Italian meal at our favorite restaurant. Over a bottle of wine or two, Carol suggested that we could celebrate completion of our goals by taking a trip. I agreed wholeheartedly because we had not traveled together, having dated only a short time, and it would be a great opportunity to get to know each other much better. As the night went on, our plans were hatched, and they evolved from the original idea of 2 weeks of camping in Colorado to our final resolve of a 6-month backpacking trip around Europe. For the next 6 months, we worked toward accomplishing our goals, noting the milestones along the way as we passed tests, wrote papers, accrued overtime, and completed classes. We kept our focus on goal completion, and 6 months after we had established those goals, we celebrated their accomplishment by departing for Europe.

Probably one of my most valued goals was my plan to propose marriage to Carol. It was February 1988, and we were 7 months into a yearlong backpacking trip around the world. We were hiking along the Jomson Trek in Nepal and had the opportunity to barter with Tibetan refugees for some jewelry made in their village. While Carol haggled over the price of bracelets, a ring caught my eye. It was very crude, gold colored, and the designs on the ring somehow seemed to be very symbolic of the Himalayas. While Carol was busy dealing with the bracelets, I paid for the ring with a pair of long johns, which I dug out of my backpack. Deal completed, we moved down the trail. The landscape at 8,900 feet was very barren, the weather very cold, and the winds ferocious.

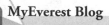

MyEverest Blog

Hey! My name is Dan, one of the students that you spoke to at Almonte High School before you left. I just wanted you to know that the stories you told to the class helped me to find what I wanted to do with my future and I hope you attain your goals as well. So get to the top Pat! And good luck! PEACE.—Dan

One week later we descended into Pokhara at 3000 feet, a small town nestled in the Himalayan mountain range, and here we took a well-deserved rest; the past few weeks of hiking in the mountains had been quite rigorous. With the sun setting in the mountains, a large white Brahman bull lying in the middle of the dirt street immediately in front of us, a candle that had been melted into the top of our crude wooden table aglow with flame, and a glass of Himalayan lager in hand, I decided it was time to propose marriage. I had pondered doing it a few times earlier in our trip: once when we were scuba diving on the Great Barrier Reef in Australia, another time when we were climbing the Great Wall of China, and the last occasion when we were riding elephants through the jungles of Northern Thailand. This place felt right because we both loved the mountains and the view was breathtaking, literally. On bent knee, I pulled out the native ring and asked Carol to marry me. She had not seen me

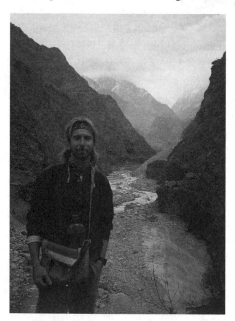

bartering for the ring and was caught by surprise. She accepted, and we had the best celebratory meal of our lives. On return to the guest house where we were staying, I mentioned to the owner that I had just proposed. His response was a cordial wish of a thousand children, to which I replied that this was a curse where I came from. Later that night a very violent earthquake actually shook us out of bed, so I like to tell people that the night I proposed to Carol I made the earth move for her. One year later, Carol jokingly gave me an opportunity to rescind my proposal because she felt that the altitude had affected my judgment. My goal had been to propose marriage, and there was no need to revisit this goal.

My Journey in Nursing

MyEverest Blog

Becoming a nurse was something I've wanted since I was a little girl. I have enjoyed my profession very much! I have done several different things and really liked them all. I was a critical care nurse in CCU for 18 years. I guess you could say I was a real adrenaline junkie. After that, I was a nursing director for Cardiac Services and Emergency Dept. (separately) for 12 years. Now, I've gone back into Cardiac/Pulmonary Rehab. We exercise both cardiac and pulmonary patients. In addition, we teach life style changes to them and their families. Really in nursing you can do so many things. You can have the drama of the ICU, a less dramatic pace in an outpatient setting, or you can do patient education. This is just a small sample of all the opportunities available to nurses. The best part is that you're always needed. :)—SD

Living, Loving, Learning, and Leaving a Legacy

Teaching has been a goal of mine for longer than I thought: I can't help but think how powerful the effects of those who teach are. It was a teacher who was able to see in me that I had what it took to be a nurse, and I have always been appreciative of her faith in me. Other teachers inspired and intrigued me to challenge myself by traveling, attaining higher education, and becoming a teacher myself. These people have had a significant effect on my life, and now I am that teacher who has the opportunity to shape lives and train our youths to be the best that they can be.

I keep a small piece of rock from the top of **Mt. Everest** on my office desk for two reasons: to remind me of the great potential that we have within us to do anything we put our minds to and also to remind me of the great responsibility I have to find that potential in my students. Many students have low self-esteem, do not realize their capacity to do well, and often need help to establish goals for their futures. I use the analogy of college as a climb up **Mt. Everest** with Base Camp being their freshman semester where they are building their support, getting their gear ready, and choosing their teammates. Camps 1, 2, 3, and 4 are synonymous with the ends of their years of college, and Summit Day is their graduation. I encourage my students to reward themselves as they gradually make it closer to their summit of education because that helps them enjoy the journey of the experience.

> **MyEverest Quote**
>
> "We will travel as far as we can, but we cannot in one lifetime see all that we would like to see or to learn all that we hunger to know."—Loren Eiseley

Tools of the Trade

To assure a safe climb to the top of a mountain, you need a wide variety of tools, such as ice ax, crampons, and harness. To reach the top of the nursing profession, you also need a variety of tools—completion of a nursing program, success in passing the NCLEX exams, and then the achievement of higher education. Attaining higher education became a realistic goal as I worked to improve myself in the clinical setting. It had been 12 years since I graduated from St. Lawrence College in Brockville, Ontario, with my degree in nursing, and I felt it was time to return to school. As I prepared for my certification test to become a certified emergency nurse (CEN), I was also a full-time student at Corpus Christi State University, where I was working on my bachelor of science in nursing. I accomplished both goals at about the same time and know that

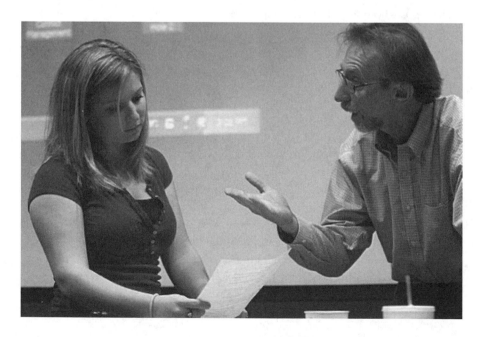

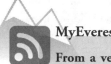

MyEverest Blog

From a very young age I knew I wanted to be a nurse. My aunt, who was a nurse, recognized this and nurtured my dreams by sewing nurses' uniforms for me when I was four and ten. The first was a student's and the second a graduate's. I have pictures of myself lovingly caring for my "patients," the dolls of all my friends. My dream was put on hold after high school and it was in my early forties that I decided the time had come to pursue it … and I am so glad that I did. Nursing has brought me so much joy and satisfaction that another profession could not. Within nursing there are so many different opportunities to explore, it is easy to find where you fit. It is so much more than paperwork, which is also computer work these days. I have worked on a medical/surgical unit with a specialty in orthopedics and neurology. Using your knowledge, skills and intuition to help patients and their families cope with diagnosis, treatment and recovery is tremendously rewarding. I now work in a pre admissions setting as part of the surgical services team and find great satisfaction in seeing that patients are properly prepared for surgery, physically and mentally. After 20 years as a nurse I still enjoy and look forward to going to the hospital each day. Though I'm planning to retire in a few years (which is why we need new nurses coming along!), I enjoy it so much that I will continue to work per diem.—J

this complemented my job as an emergency room charge nurse. Twelve years later I returned to school again, this time to earn a master of science in health education from the University of South Carolina. This degree again supported my role as an operating room educator and gave me the tools to better educate my new nurses as they oriented to the perioperative setting. Through my role as an educator in the operating room, I also scheduled observation days for BSN nursing students and truly enjoyed exposing them to a variety of surgical scenarios.

I sought a master's degree not only to support my role as an educator, but to teach at the university level. During the summer of my master's degree graduation, I obtained adjunct faculty status in the College of Nursing at the University of South Carolina. I taught a perioperative surgical elective to BSN nursing students and loved it! I inquired about teaching at the university level there and was told by a seasoned faculty member that I should pursue a doctoral degree. I immediately applied and was accepted into a doctoral program. Three years later, I graduated from the University of South Carolina with a doctorate in public health.

With the new degree in hand, I left my hospital job and started teaching full time. However, in order to comply with a state board of nursing regulation that required faculty members have either their master's or doctorate in nursing, I began my new role as a faculty member while attending classes for a master's degree. Two years later, I graduated with my master's in nursing. Having what you need, when you need it, is vital to the success of any plan, whether it be acquiring higher education, teaching a class of nursing students, changing a dressing on a patient, or climbing up the side of a mountain.

MyEverest Blog

I read that the Sherpas believe that the mountain allows those with a just cause to be successful in the summit attempt. I can't think of anyone with a cause that is more just than yours. "Enjoy when you can and endure when you must." Johann Wolfgang von Goethe. —SD

My Climbs on the Mountains

In 1993, after years of planning, my wife and I backpacked through Latin America for an entire year. We began by boarding a Greyhound bus from Columbia, South Carolina, to Corpus Christi, Texas, where we visited friends before our short drive to the border of Mexico. At this stage, "where the rubber meets the road," we walked across the United States–Mexico border to start a journey with no specific destination. Spontaneity, a desire for adventure, and a willingness to try just about anything once, twice if we liked it, was the theme for our yearlong trip. This aptitude to experiment and to challenge ourselves led to many exciting adventures that would fill an entire series of books.

One of those chance happenings occurred while we were visiting Baños, Ecuador. We had left the United States 6 months earlier, and it was time now to purchase some better outerwear because the basic gear we had brought was not adequate for the frequent exposure to wind and rain. While shopping in an outdoor gear shop, I happened to notice a group of young men and women bartering with the store owner, a common sight in Latin America. At times we would walk away from the interaction, only to have the store owner come after us to offer an even lower acceptable price, which was probably still 100% profit for the dealer.

Those who bartered longest usually did better, and this seemed to be the case with this group, because the owner continued to offer lower prices and the group continued to haggle more. As I passed within earshot, I heard the group excitedly discussing renting gear and acquiring a guiding service for a climb on a local mountain. It was just at that moment that one of the group members turned to me, apparently interpreting my look as one of interest in their haggling, and asked me a question that would forever change my life: "Hey you, do you want to join us to climb a mountain?"

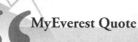

MyEverest Quote

"Kind words can be short and easy to speak, but their echoes are truly endless."—Mother Teresa

Creating a Larger Vision for Life

Before that day, I had been a hiker and camper and always enjoyed the mountain vistas, but not once had I ever considered standing on top of one! I cast a glance at Carol for approval/disapproval, but she was busy shopping, so with little hesitation (save for a long deep breath), I replied, "Sure, why not." It is funny how the most inconspicuous moments can be so dynamic and life-changing. The climbing terminology was new to me, and the gear even more so, because I had never, ever pondered the possibility of so grand an adventure. Up until that moment, the highest that I had ever been was at the top of the Eiffel Tower, and that was a major challenge because of my debilitating fear of heights. On that day in Paris, at the top of the tower, my wife had to literally unglue me from the elevator's back wall so that I could take in the view of Paris spread out below us. I can't remember much of that view because my fear had paralyzed me so that I could see only far distances, but I have heard that it is spectacular.

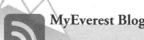

MyEverest Blog

Keep your head on straight—safety before glory.—DG

Once the decision was made, much to the concern of my wife, things happened very rapidly. I was quickly fitted with high-tech clothing—which included Gore-Tex pants and jacket, fleece top and bottoms, boots that made me think I was going skiing, and an assortment of gloves, socks, and hats—all designed for warmth and efficiency.

The fitting took minutes, but the process was lasting because I was now entering a world that was totally unknown to me. Never in my wildest dreams had I imagined this scenario! This dream that I had never had became a reality when a few days later I was driving up to the biggest mountain I had ever seen. On the way to Base Camp, our guide helped us to acclimatize to the altitude by leading us through an exhausting workout of jumping jacks along the trail, an exercise that I later found to be futile.

In our high camp, at 12,000 feet, we fixed our last meal and settled into bunks to obtain much-needed sleep; however, it evaded us: nervousness and fear of the unknown gave rise to anxiety and even nausea. One of our group members succumbed to the high altitude and became incapacitated by severe headaches and uncontrollable vomiting. At midnight we exited camp, dressed in high-tech clothing, and were challenged immediately by a heavy snowstorm. A few hours later we reached the glacier field, and it was here that we put crampons on our boots to give us better stability and connected ourselves to each other by rope and harness. This connectivity, and the fact that we had practiced emergency and life-saving procedures, gave me a false sense of security. However, the thought of arresting a tumble into a crevasse by falling onto the ground and jamming an ice ax into the snow was not very comforting.

Risks That Changed the Direction of My Life

The storm had now intensified, and visibility was down to a few feet. It was getting much more difficult to look straight ahead due to the blinding snow driven by escalating winds, yet we continued to climb. Gray shadows along the trail materialized into deep, dark, yawning crevasses that threatened to swallow us, should we step outside of the footprint tracked in the snow by the climber in front of us. Halfway up the mountain, we encountered two groups of climbers being driven back by the weather. Our guide continued, undaunted by the storm raging all around us. It was soon thereafter that another person in our group began to show symptoms of cerebral edema: he complained of headaches, which were then followed by nausea and vomiting. A support guide escorted him off the mountain while we continued upward.

MyEverest Quote

"As in any alpine region, the weather is changeable, protection questionable, route-finding bewildering, rockfall frequent and descents tedious. In short, it's everything you could ever ask for."—*Canadian Alpine Journal*, 1993

About 4:00 AM the storm broke, and we were treated with the most beautiful view of the lights of Quito, Ecuador. It was at this moment that I suddenly realized how high we had climbed already and how fearful of heights I was! Looking down always does it to me. As night turned to day, we found ourselves on the final approach. The air was thin, we gasped for each breath, and our leg muscles burned with the exertion of climbing straight upward. This was not fun; this was a challenge. And to make matters worse, the view all around me was nauseating because all I could see was how far I could fall, should I slip or trip. How did I get here? Why was I on this mountain? Who were these maniacs that I was strapped to? At 9:00 AM, we took the last few steps that were to become my first training steps onto the roof of Ecuador. What a relief, what a view, what an accomplishment! I was hooked!

On that day I dug pretty deep and pushed myself to a level that I had never been before. I believe that we nurses dig deep each and every day as we are challenged with the crevasses in the hospital, the height of the challenge, the energy that it takes to accomplish the enormity of the task, and the lack of resources that causes excess stress. To date it was the most challenging thing that I had ever done, and the exhilaration of standing on top of this mountain was something that I had never experienced in my life. I had triumphed over my asthmatic condition and proved to myself the old adage that if there is a will, there is a way.

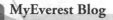

MyEverest Blog

I have been run over, kicked, bitten, stomped, reared up with and bucked by many horses. Why do I keep riding, because when it all clicks, it's the best and I feel alive. I understand why you climb.—MB

This random event of personal challenge fired within me a desire to challenge myself again on a mountain, so on my return home from our yearlong trip through Latin America, I started to climb Colorado's "fourteeners." There are 54 mountains in Colorado that are over 14,000 feet, and all are challenging in their own right. Now that I was starting to get used to higher altitudes, I needed to get experience on snowfields and glaciers. Weather and conditioning were my biggest obstacles during my climb and summit of **Mt. Rainier** (14,410 feet) in Washington State. This climb tested my ability to endure cold weather, snow, and glacial travel as well as my capacity to function as a member of a climbing team. I was literally on an emotional high after my summit of **Mt. Rainier** but still felt the need to challenge myself further.

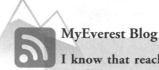

MyEverest Blog

I know that reaching the summit is not a given, but a hard and carefully earned achievement. —MH

Beginning With the End in Mind

And then it happened, a disaster on **Mt. Everest**. It was May 1996 when eight climbers were killed near the top of **Mt. Everest** as they encountered a blizzard that left them stranded in harsh conditions. One of the survivors, Beck Weathers, suffered severe frostbite and had to have amputation of both his right arm below the elbow and all fingers and thumb of his left hand. Beck also had to have his nose amputated and

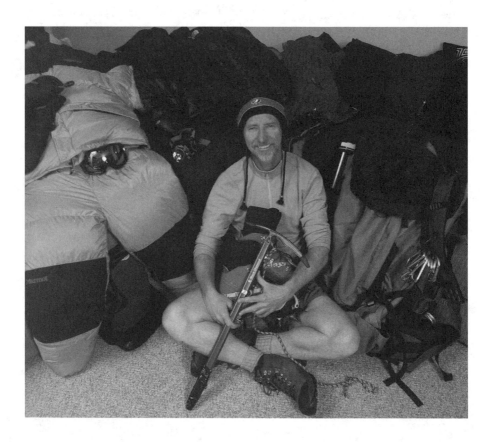

reconstructed. His ordeal, and that of his climbing team, was made famous by Jon Krakauer's best-selling book, *Into Thin Air*. As the tragedy unfolded in newspapers, magazines, television, and Internet-based mountaineering Web sites, I remember my shock that such tragedy could happen to experienced climbers. One of those stories mentioned that if Beck had completed his summit of **Mt. Everest**, he would have fulfilled his quest to climb the "7 Summits of the World."

This was the first time that I had heard of the "7 Summits of the World" and was intrigued to learn more. I found that they were the 7 highest mountains on the 7 continents of the world and had been climbed by fewer than 100 people. Further research revealed that these summits had taken many lives and were not for the faint of heart. The conditions would be challenging, access to the mountains problematic, and the unknowns of the climbs outnumbered the known. These three factors were instrumental in my decision to climb the "7 Summits of the World," because the challenge would take me outside of my comfort zone into an unfamiliar area of expertise.

MyEverest Blog

7 Summits: that's like winning the Nextel Cup, Super Bowl, Stanley Cup and the lottery all at once!!—Ken

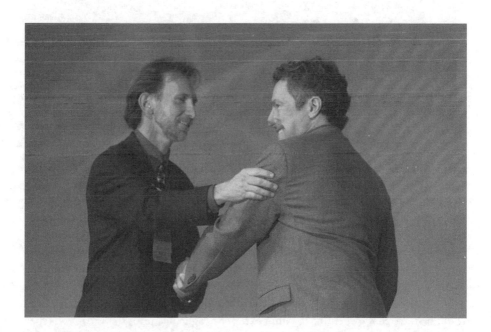

It was both scary and exciting to set a goal of climbing the "7 Summits of the World" in 7 years. The actual planning for the 7 Summits became somewhat similar to a business plan because in order to accomplish my lofty goal, I had to do a lot of research, undergo extensive physical training, plan transportation and guides, and establish extensive time-lines—all of this around a full schedule of school, work, and, of course, personal life.

I met Beck in Dallas in 2001, when I introduced him as our keynote speaker at the annual conference of the Association of periOperative Registered Nurses (AORN). Beck was our motivational speaker, and that afternoon there was not a dry eye in the convention hall as Beck relived that fateful night on **Mt. Everest** when he lost so many of his close friends. I told Beck that night that his plight had inspired me to some degree to pursue the same challenge he had chosen; however, in doing so I hoped to become the first nurse to complete the "7 Summits of the World." Beck was supportive of my dream, and when he autographed the inside cover of his book, *Left for Dead*, he wrote me these encouraging words: "Climb High."

MyEverest Blog

You continue in our thoughts and prayers as you approach the summit. Thank you for the example you have set for the students in the USC Nursing program! You have instilled in them the value of setting goals and reaching beyond themselves.
—Anonymous

Letting Go of the Past

Another goal involved a commitment to a friend, Sean Egan. When I discovered in 2004 that my hometown friend, Sean, was planning to climb **Mt. Everest**, I was elated! At that time, I had climbed four of the 7 Summits of the World and felt I could change the sequence of remaining mountains to climb **Mt. Everest** in 2005 with Sean. It would be so special to have two people from the same town climb **Mt. Everest** together. Sean and I had talked mountaineering for years; he had already been to **Mt. Everest** Base Camp to do research and had wondered aloud about the possibility of going higher on the mountain. Sean had already explored the Khumbu Icefall and was excited about the chance to move farther up the mountain. Initially, I was able to make the required changes in home, school, and work life to be able to join Sean on his team, but soon thereafter I realized that I could not go and we would not be able to climb together. In the meantime, Sean continued to give me training tips and shared with me his mantra, *Festina Lente*, which is Latin for "take it slow and easy." I encouraged Sean to get some altitude and cold-weather experience, and as a result he traveled to Argentina to climb **Mt. Aconcagua** just prior to his trip to Nepal!

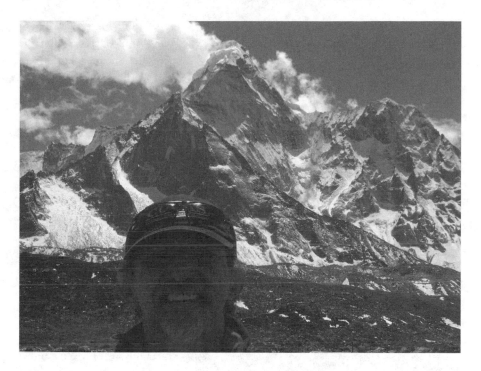

In spring 2005, I was able to keep in touch with Sean via e-mail while he climbed **Mt. Everest**. When he got sick, I remember advising him to go lower on the mountain to recuperate. Days later, I was stunned to find out that he had died while trying to recuperate! I couldn't believe it! Carol was out of town when I heard of Sean's death, and I remember when she came home how I told her, between sobs, that Sean had died. I can't remember the last time I cried, but I did that night. I called Sean's climbing partner Harold soon thereafter and told him that Sean had started the trail to the top for me, and that I planned to finish the journey for both of us! In spring 2007, I contacted Sean's daughter, Anna, and she gave me a small urn with Sean's ashes in it so he could "join me for the journey." I made plans at that time to release his ashes at the top of **Mt. Everest**, where we would finish our journey "together."

MyEverest Blog

Knew you could do it. I am so proud of you and your courageous goals. Walk careful coming down. Your friend's spirit was with you all the way. You were indeed a true friend. All the power and money in the world cannot buy true friendship, it is given. Bless you and enjoy the accomplishment.—Anonymous

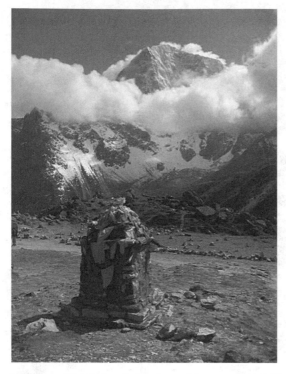

On my initial walk in to Base Camp, I came upon the memorial shrine (chorten) in Sean's honor, and it caught me by surprise. The view of Awi Peak from his shrine is breathtaking and is a very serene site amidst the other memorial shrines that represent the great number of fellow climbers who have died on **Mt. Everest**. Visiting Sean's memorial site reinforced my need and desire to get to the top of **Mt. Everest** so we could both finish the adventure. As if the climb on Summit Day were not challenging enough, I now had a self-imposed pressure to finish the climb for myself—and a friend who lived in spirit only.

I had promised Carol that I would turn around if there were any problems, stop if I had any doubts, and retreat if there were any questions of safety, but what of my promise to Sean?

I had silently prayed that I would continue our journey, finish the trip, and by doing so bring closure to 2 years of grief over his untimely death. The weight of the urn in my backpack grew heavier as I approached the summit, and I felt the pressure to keep going, despite all! On that summit bid, I spoke to Sean quite a lot and actually cursed him for being so heavy, both on my heart and my mind. Maybe it was the guilt of not being with him in 2005, and the knowledge that I might have been able to save his life. Perhaps it was the desire to have him there with me. And then, I was there, on top of the world: we had made it! After a few photos by Dhorjee, my Sherpa, I decided it was time to release Sean's ashes. I tried to explain to Dhorjee what I was about to do, but his English was very limited, and after a minute or so he simply walked away from me, leaving me totally alone on top of the world! I took advantage of this solo time to release Sean's ashes, and with great ease those ashes were lifted high on the raging winds and spread across a wide expanse of mountainous land, just as Sean would have liked it! What a view, what a place, and what a great time to have this momentous occasion! After releasing the ashes, I repeated a quote that had been sent to me from Sandra Dickson, a nurse colleague and friend in Columbia.

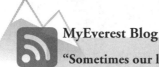

MyEverest Blog

"Sometimes our light goes out but is blown into flame by another human being. Each of us owes deepest thanks to those who have rekindled this light." Albert Schweitzer.—SD

Sean's memory has been kept alive by those closest to him. He made a major difference in people's lives and continues to do so: a school has been built in Kathmandu as a lasting tribute to his legacy. Now our journey is complete, and mission accomplished. If only we could have stood on the summit together … but then again, we did!

Table 4-1   Goals Checklist

Review the following list to see how many goals you have established in life.

Goal Setting	Yes	No
Personal		
• Write down goals		
• Categorize goals		
• Set all goals with a timeline		
• Troubleshoot potential challenges to goals		
• Change routines to achieve goals		
• Know goals of significant others		
• Focus on goals and see self achieving them and enjoying success		
• Revisit goals regularly to update		
• Add new goals once others are completed		
• Have plan should you fail to complete goal		
• Have motivation to accomplish goals		
• Am prepared to break routines to accomplish goals		
Academic		
• Have developed educational/career goals		
• Take responsibility for my academic success		
• Know goals of worksite/school		
• Am an active, not passive student		

Chapter 5
Attitude

Charles Shultz's Philosophy

1. Name the five wealthiest people in the world.
2. Name the last five Heisman trophy winners.
3. Name the last five winners of the Miss America contest.
4. Name 10 people who have won the Nobel or Pulitzer Prize.
5. Name the last dozen Academy Award winners for best actor and actress.
6. Name the last decade's worth of World Series winners.

How did you do? The point is, none of us remember the headliners of yesterday. These are no second-rate achievers. They are the best in their fields. But the applause dies. Awards tarnish. Achievements are forgotten. Accolades and certificates are buried with their owners.

Here's another quiz:

1. List a few teachers who aided your journey through school.
2. Name three friends who have helped you through a difficult time.
3. Name five people who have taught you something worthwhile.
4. Think of a few people who have made you feel appreciated and special.
5. Think of five people you enjoy spending time with.
6. Name half a dozen heroes whose stories have inspired you.

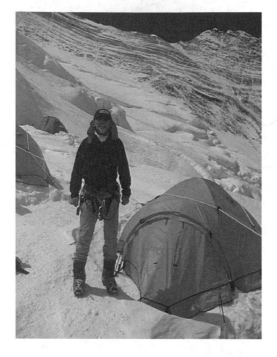

Easier? The lesson: The people who make a difference in your life are not those with the most credentials, the most money, or the most awards. They are the ones who care!

What is attitude, and why is it so important? Where do we learn attitude, and when learned can we change it? According to Merriam-Webster's Collegiate Dictionary, 11th edition, *attitude* is "a mental position with regard to a fact or state," or "a feeling or emotion toward a fact or state." One only has to Google the word *attitude* to receive a resounding 116,000,000 results. Listed are attitude quotes, the powers of attitude, attitude definitions, tips on attitude, tools to change your attitude, mothers with attitude, cheeky attitude, and many sites listing attitude associated with sports and diseases. A search of the term *attitude books* netted a mere 25,900,000 results with themes dealing with how to build, change, and adopt attitudes in both our personal and work lives. With all of these resources and information, one would think that everyone should have a winning positive attitude, but we know that is not the case! In both our personal and our work lives we interface on a daily basis with many people who have less than adequate attitudes and at times can transfer their bad attitudes to us. In a recent poll, mental attitude was rated highest as the key to happiness, yet why is it so lacking in our environments? Sometimes in the daily challenges that life gives us, we miss what is really important. We may fail to say hello, please, or thank you, congratulate someone on something wonderful that has happened to him or her, give a compliment, or just do something nice for no reason.

MyEverest Blog

"Follow your passion for it will take you far beyond your everyday life."—MC

One thing that has always surprised me has been the question, both before and after my summit of **Mt. Everest**, asked by quite a lot of people: "Are you going all the way to the top?" I have always been surprised by this question and never quite understood the significance until recently. I believe that for most **Mt. Everest** represents the most challenging physical quest on this planet and is something that takes a superhuman effort that can be attempted only by a select few. Additionally, many of the movies and television shows that depict **Mt. Everest** climbs show the extreme conditions and the tragedy that can and does occur. So, it is no wonder that most are surprised to meet someone who is planning to climb to the top of the world. But then there is the question of going all the way to the top. I can easily understand the concerns of extreme cold and tragedy, but why would I want to go only part way to the top?

> **MyEverest Quote**
>
> **"In the confrontation between the stream and the rock, the stream always wins—not through strength, but by perseverance."**
> —H. Jackson Brown

To use an analogy in our school setting, would a student seek to complete only a portion of a degree program and not try to graduate? I have come to believe, though, that most people's concern is related to the feared danger associated with the final push to the top and not the capacity to make that push. I have used these analogies to help my students understand that they need to prepare well for the final push for graduation and never relax or let down their guards.

My Travels Through Life

My wife Carol has been the one who has helped me to see that the journey through life, as opposed to the destination, is most important. As I began my quest to climb the 7 Summits of the World, I was juggling full-time work, with transitions from staff to management positions, and was a full-time university student working on completion of three back-to-back degrees: a master of science in health education, a doctorate in public health, and a master's in nursing. My focus while in school was graduating with a degree, whereas on the mountain it was getting to the summit. However, I found that solely focusing on the end result was disappointing because the degree became just a piece of framed paper on my office wall, and the summit became just that, another summit. Carol helped me understand that I should not be so focused on success because if I didn't slow down and enjoy the journey, I would miss out on some valuable

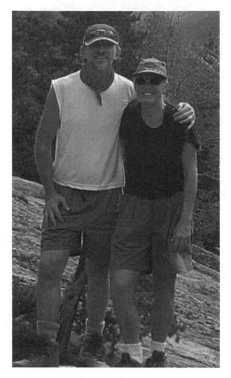

experiences. The journey then became my focus, and I began to enjoy even more the camaraderie of students and climbers, the thrill of academic and climbing challenges, and the satisfaction of a job well done. This focus was reinforced on **Mt. Everest** as I made my final push to the summit. Carol sought reassurance that if problems developed, I would turn around and abate my summit bid. She reinforced for me that there was more to life than standing on top of the world and that she wanted to spend the rest of her life with me in person, not lamenting my loss on a failed attempt.

What Motivates You

However, it was my motivation to climb and challenge myself that really gave my life meaning. I have observed many colleagues who have burned out and left our profession because they felt that their efforts in helping people were no longer meaningful. Keeping motivated is a big challenge. I have found that motivation can be accomplished by dreaming of the future, selecting positive role models, mentoring those who want to learn, and all the while enjoying the journey. Many people start their day by worrying about the problems, people, and challenges that they will encounter, instead of looking forward to the people they will met and the opportunities to accomplish tasks, despite the barriers. Life is, after all, what you make of it. The more you put into it, the more it reflects back on you.

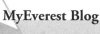

MyEverest Blog

This is likely my first and only post, just not into it, for the most part, but wanted to congratulate you on your successes. I have been following your climb and have found your posts to be informative and motivational. From you posts it is evident that your relationship with Carol is special and in today's world somewhat unique. Makes sure you enjoy one another as life is too short for anything else. I suspect Everest has reinforced this for you.—H

A positive attitude is vital not only in the work setting, but in our daily lives, and even more important when we travel because sometimes the worst of conditions can bring out the worst in us. While backpacking around the world for a year in 1988, we were exposed to many deplorable conditions, and all required a positive attitude because everywhere we went we were ambassadors for our countries. One situation that stands out occurred in Northern Thailand, where we were visiting the Karen tribespeople. During a weeklong trek through the jungles, we visited one village where we were given accommodations in a palm-thatched hut, directly over a pigsty. Meals were cooked within the hut, with smoke escaping through the cracks in the walls because there was no other ventilation. The smell of smoke, mixed with the stench of pigs, created an overwhelming effect that had us staggering around the camp. This turned out to be one of our most special experiences because the native people opened their village to us, and it was our positive attitudes, despite very primitive conditions, that led them to befriend us.

My Journey in Nursing

MyEverest Blog

"The reward is not in the acknowledgement of helping a fellow human being; it is in the act itself."—MC

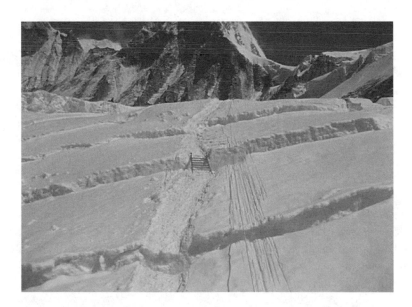

To use a mountaineering analogy regarding attitude, I like to speak of the crevasses that we experience in our workplace settings. On the mountains, a *crevasse* is a glacier fracture that may be a wide and gaping hole that is difficult to transit and/or could be covered by a snow bridge and not easily seen. Both are a danger to mountaineers: one easily seen and the other a danger lurking just below the surface. The crevasses that we deal with in our personal lives and at work are the personalities, egos, and attitudes that sometimes are counterproductive, as well as the hectic pace, resultant mistakes, and, of course, all the other stressors.

In the medical setting, we need to ask ourselves, if we already know where those crevasses are located, how do we avoid falling into them? We also need to be prepared for a tumble into a "workplace crevasse" because we need to know how to get out, and who and where our support systems are that can help us. As with the crevasses on the mountains, sometimes we can see people who have what we consider a negative attitude, yet at other times we see people whose negative attitude lies just below the surface and can break through without warning. We need to prevent circumstances from controlling our destiny and put ourselves in control, whether at school as a student, at work as a nurse, or on the mountain as a climber.

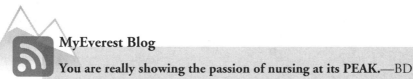

MyEverest Blog

You are really showing the passion of nursing at its PEAK.—BD

Attitude Is Everything

Attitudes are the ways of responding to people and situations that we have learned based on our beliefs and value systems. These attitudes are then manifested through our behaviors. In nursing, a positive attitude is indispensable to proper patient care. However, we vary quite considerably in our attitudes toward our patients, who can be comprised of rapists, substance abusers, child molesters, and those involved in other deviant behaviors, as well as patients who are incarcerated, suffer from mental illness, have a transmissible infectious disease, and those who a have terminal disease. We vary in our attitudes toward complementary and alternative medicine, spirituality, technology, death and dying, and even our ability to help a patient deal with pain. On a personal level, our attitudes all vary significantly regarding work, life, age, gender, race, and ethnicity. These attitudes have been developed through exposure to our families, friends, and life events. In every patient contact, our attitude affects quality healthcare delivery.

MyEverest Blog

Hey Pat—glad to hear your decathlon (of its own customized definition) is coming to an end. But I am wondering what sort of let down you might have upon return. It will be difficult to truly absorb all that you have experienced—and there is not a bigger mountain to accomplish (what to do from here?!). As you have said in the past, it began as a midlife crisis—so perhaps, the crisis has also been left behind (as has the midlife—huh?). As we continue on into the 50s, at least for me, I have different perspective from the 30s and 40s. But then, I may not push myself like you do—perhaps you will have more adventures you are striving for (but what can "top" Everest?!). I trust you are journaling all that you have experienced emotionally and spiritually—as your journey is not one that is superficial (even though, physiologically it must ache and hurt superficially as well!). Guess it is called "all consuming."—BD

Attitude adjustment has become a buzzword in our work settings and is most often typified by corporate getaways, unit parties, team-building exercises, and happy hours at bars where alcohol consumption and its ability to change bad attitudes have become quite popular. Collectively as nurses our attitudes also vary toward technology, men in nursing, physicians, and even our health team members. A negative outcome of these attitudinal differences is a recently named syndrome that has been around for some time: *lateral violence*, which is defined by the International Council of Nurses as "behavior that humiliates, degrades, or otherwise indicates a lack of respect for the dignity and worth of an individual." Many nursing groups have taken a stand on this issue: the Center for American Nurses position states, "there is no place in a professional practice environment for lateral violence and bullying among nurses or between healthcare professionals," and the Council on Surgical and Perioperative Safety states, "violence or the threat of violence in the workplace must not be tolerated in any circumstance. The creation of a violence-free culture of mutual respect, dignity and fairness among individuals and professional disciplines is essential for the teamwork and communication necessary for patient safety."

MyEverest Blog

"Be the inspiration that you seek from others."—MC

Attitude Is a Choice

We decide what attitude we will adopt in any given situation, but at work it seems like we are not making the right choices. I like to use the crayon analogy. Imagine a box of crayons: some are sharp, some are pretty, some are dull, and some have weird names—and all are different colors. But they all have to live in the same box. The message here is that we don't necessarily have to love one another, but we do have to get along!

When I worked as an assistant nurse manager in the operating room at Palmetto Health Richland in Columbia, my job was that of a board runner. This position was like that of an air traffic controller: every day I managed an overscheduled list of surgical cases, surgeons, nurses, and surgical techs, add-on emergent cases, and only a limited number of rooms and equipment. Surgical cases had to be delayed to make room for emergencies, and staff had to be moved around like chess pieces to a surgical case that matched their expertise. Each day started with a packed schedule that often "went to hell in a handbasket" because all it took was for one person to call in sick and/or one case to go longer than the assigned time to cause a disruption in the schedule.

MyEverest Blog

"Patience is seeing the big picture and knowing it is worth it."—MC

My day started earlier than most because it was my responsibility to trouble-shoot the schedule, make the daily assignments, and have everything in order before the staff started walking out of the lounge at about 6:30 AM. Because the schedule could change at a moment's notice, a lot of the staff felt great unease as they arrived each day: there was always uncertainty about what their day would be like. Most people looked upon it as a challenge, and all were able to step up to that challenge when it did occur; however, there were a select few who started each day with a scowl on their face, as they ambled slowly to the desk to see what their assignment was for that day. A quick review of the assignment was usually accompanied by loud moans and groans and a resignation that this day would be the worst that they ever had. This negativity had a way of infecting others: over time, I noticed that those who moaned and groaned each day had multiplied and the chorus of discontent was spreading.

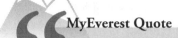

Building an A-Team

In consultation with the management team, we decided to try to develop a more positive attitude among our staff. We felt that we were not as visible as we could be in the midst of the daily work routines, so assistant nurse manager desks were moved out of offices and strategically placed into the middle of corridors closest to their specialty teams and equipment. Daily work schedules began to reflect the management team's involvement in surgical cases as they began to both circulate and scrub in on cases to start the day and then daily began relieving their team members during the lunch break. As the board runner, and first member of the management team whom the staff saw each day, I felt that it was important for me to set the tone and help promote a positive attitude among our staff.

Each day as the staff approached the desk, I would greet them with a smile and cheery words of encouragement. At times, I would wear a comical mask to lighten the mood and on occasion would chase staff down the hall that refused to smile or laugh at my antics. Some would even try to get to their assigned rooms without passing by the front desk, and in doing so avoid having a management-imposed attitude adjustment. However, my early morning rounds took me through each of the operating rooms so for those who did not get an early morning attitude adjustment, there was a mid-morning adjustment ready to help get them through the day. The end of the day always proved to be a pressure cooker because there were always more cases running at change of shift than we had staff to manage the rooms. Again management stepped up to maintain the positive attitude that was now taking over the hectic work environment and began to stay late and help complete the cases. This action allowed staff to get home on time, kids to be picked up from school, appointments kept, and errands completed. Additionally, those staff that volunteered to stay late were given days off and/or allowed to leave early on another day or come in a little later. The combination of all these efforts, collectively on behalf of management and the staff, helped people to develop a much more positive attitude within our work setting. This shift in attitude helped to promote the willingness of staff members to seek leadership positions because they wanted to be a part of a progressive team. To truly lead and make a difference in our world, we need to start with ourselves, and be an example to those with whom we work. Don't be the type of person who waits to be told to do something—just do it!

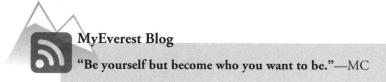

MyEverest Blog

"Be yourself but become who you want to be."—MC

My Climbs on the Mountains

I have been impressed with all the climbers I have met over the years; almost all have had a "take no prisoners" approach to accomplishing the task at hand. This adventurous attitude is critical to succeeding in life, whether it be the challenge of a climb or the opportunity to "think outside the box" at work.

What It Takes to Get to the Top

It was August 2002 and we were visiting Washington State with a group of friends as we had planned to climb to the summit of **Mt. Baker**. At a height of almost 11,000 feet it does not appear to be a formidable challenge, but its route to the top is quite deceiving as it is crisscrossed with snow, glaciers, and crevasses. The hike to high-camp challenged our fitness regimen, yet our spirits remained high as we established camp during a light afternoon snowfall. Later, nestled in our sleeping bags, we tried to rest in anticipation of a late night departure. However, the sounds of accelerating wind and heavy snow sliding off our tent roofs gave way to feelings of concern as the weather was suddenly becoming a factor that we had not anticipated. With the departure hour approaching, our 3-person team exited the camp into what had become an almost blinding snowstorm. No problem, I thought, as this is what mountaineering is all about. Climbing a mountain without challenges would be too easy, and if it were so easy wouldn't everyone be doing it? Or so I thought!

As we left the warmth of tents and friends, we slowly headed straight upward at a very severe angle and within minutes our pace had slowed to very deliberate steps in the snow as our leader blazed a trail. Snow whipped up by the wind continued to challenge our positive attitudes, as somehow this cold precipitation began to penetrate our layers of protective clothing and found its way to exposed tissue. The bite of the wind was sharp, and if it were not for our Gore-Tex balaclava facemasks we would be soon suffering from frostbite. Our headlamps cut through the dark and all we could see ahead was the white of snow falling. However, behind us there had been a solo headlamp illuminating the trail that seemed with time to be catching up to our measured pace.

It was now 1:00 AM; we had been climbing for 2 hours and the direction of snow falling on the trail had turned from a slight angle to almost parallel to the surface. The intensity of the wind had increased to a level where we could barely hear each other speak when face to face. Our leader decided that we had better turn around and return to camp. It was at this moment that the solo headlight-bearing climber caught up to us, as he had been tracking our route through the snow. We quickly made introductions and discussed our options, at which time I decided to continue up the mountain with this climber whom I had just met, while my team returned to the warmth and security of high camp.

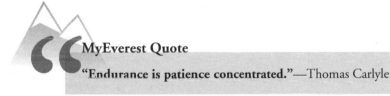

MyEverest Quote

"Endurance is patience concentrated."—Thomas Carlyle

I felt satisfaction and security because I was now climbing this mountain with a local veteran climber, and this knowledge helped to booster my waning positive attitude. As we continued upward, we followed a path that was lined with small wands bearing tiny, brightly colored pieces of cloth. Our climb turned into a game of connect the dots; we childishly looked for the next flag, and then the next, as we tried to outsmart each other regarding the direction of the route. Never once did we think about the original placement of these wands, and never did we think that they were leading us anywhere but directly, and safely, to the top of the mountain.

By 4:00 AM, the snowfall had intensified so that we could only see a few feet on either side of us. Imagine our surprise when at this moment we saw the glare of headlamps above us coming down the mountain. Within minutes, we were joined by a group of six climbers, all tethered together by rope, clothes layered in heavy snow, and faces covered entirely by balaclavas. The leader greeted us as best could be despite the roar of the wind and questioned why we were not roped together as we were in the middle of a huge field of crevasses. His parting suggestion was for us turn around just like his team had done because of the worsening weather. As they descended, I noticed that the leader was picking up the wands that had marked the trail. These were their trail markers, and we now had no way to navigate to the summit.

While we re-energized with water and energy bars, I decided to find out more about this local veteran climber, because forging forward in this crevasse field required a deep level of trust and reliance on each other's skills. What I found out next I will never, ever forget: this veteran climber was not a veteran, nor was he a local, and to make matters worse, this was his first climb on a mountain! I could not believe what I was hearing and actually had him repeat these comments. This was a potential death sentence, because this climber had no skills other than the ability to climb straight up. How could this be happening to me? I was now the veteran climber, yet still a rookie myself. I did not know this mountain and had put blind faith in a stranger who had befriended and misled me in his zealous attempt to get to the top.

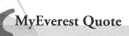

MyEverest Quote

"With ordinary talent and extraordinary perseverance, all things are attainable."—Sir Thomas Foxwell Buxton

What to do, what to do? I couldn't believe this was happening! The first thing I had to do was establish that we were safe, so I quickly roped us to each other. Next it was a matter of instructing my new acquaintance on how to arrest a fall into a crevasse and how to rescue oneself and each other should we fall. As I would, in my role as a nurse educator, I had this climber do a return demonstration to reassure me that he understood. After all, it was not only his life but now mine that he had in his hands, and vice versa. We took our time with these critical lessons, and once I felt somewhat secure I decided that it was time for us to move, and our direction would be down! However, the winds had intensified even more as we turned to descend so I decided to stay in that spot and conserve energy and warmth. As we huddled together, I started to notice grey areas around us as the ebb and flow of the winds and snow allowed momentary glimpses of our surroundings. In one particular gust the gray color turned to black, and I could clearly see that only a few feet away from our perch was the edge of a deep, cavernous crevasse so huge that an 18-wheeler truck could drive through it sideways. The futility of our situation now hit me like a sucker punch to the chin.

It was at that moment that I heard a noise with which I was not familiar. A crackling noise, and voices? Were there others around us in the storm? The noise continued and I kept looking around for other headlights. Had the climbers we previously met come back for us? As the wind abated for a moment, I again heard the voice and recognized it as Carol's! I then realized that I had a walkie-talkie deep in my down jacket that we had brought along for emergency situations but never thought would be used! I dug deep for the walkie-talkie and as I removed it from the protection of my jacket I could clearly hear the terror in Carol's voice. I quickly depressed the send button and confirmed that we were safe, yet stranded. It was now 6:00 AM and the team that I had started up the mountain with had just got into high camp, because they too had been stranded by the conditions and had to bivouac in their backpacks. They had reported to Carol was that I was lost on the mountain, not news that she wanted to hear. After I reassured Carol as best I could, despite the fact that I myself was quite scared, I spoke to my friends who had returned to camp. Their recommendation was to slowly and safely descend and to try to retrace our route. This was easier said than done, because the heavy snows had covered our tracks and there were no wands left to guide the way.

As the falling snow abated somewhat and the winds decreased to a level where we could see what lay ahead, we slowly began our torturous route down the mountain. Shapes took form and we found ourselves amidst huge towering walls of snow, with deep unforgiving crevasses crisscrossing our route. To have descended straight down would have been perilous. A few hours into our descent, we came across tents that belonged to those that had passed us in the night. It was 8:00 AM, and we woke them from a deep sleep to ask which route to take to get back to our high camp. After they gave us directions, we said good-bye and continued to slowly navigate our way as once again the snow began to fall. The landmarks were unfamiliar, each towering wall of snow looked the same as the last, yet each crevasse looked more forbidding.

The 11:00 AM hour approached, and we had now been climbing and descending for the past 12 hours. I was ready for this to be over! During the descent, we communicated with the group extensively by walkie-talkie, and it seemed like we were headed in the right direction. As we neared the camp, the snow again intensified, and we resorted to yelling as loud as we could with hopes of being heard and guided to safety. Within 30 minutes of yelling above the noise of the wind, our friends heard our voices and guided us back to camp, much the same way an air traffic controller directs a plane safely onto a runway. A prettier site I had never seen than when Carol greeted me at the camp. Feeling weathered, dehydrated, and hypothermic were the least of my worries, because I was now safely back in camp. My adventurous attitude had definitely been tested, and I learned many lessons that day, the most important of which was that getting down can be a major challenge.

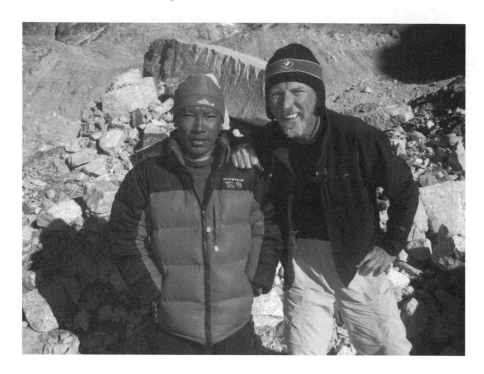

MyEverest Quote

"Courage is never to let your actions be influenced by your fears."—Arthur Koestle

Getting Down Is a Major Challenge

When I researched **Mt. Everest**, I found many pieces of information that proved to be helpful and a lot of data that was very alarming. Through years of accident investigation, it had been determined that about 80% of those who die on **Mt. Everest** do so on the journey down the mountain from the summit. These deaths were attributed to exhaustion, severe weather, hypothermia, hypoxia, and a lack of team support. And now here I was at Camp 4, just having had the most challenging day and night of my life with another legendary challenge ahead to go from Camp 4 to Base Camp.

Sometime during the night my oxygen again ran out on me, and I awoke to a flurry of activity: oxygen tanks were being replaced, Sherpas were barking at us to get out of the tents as they were being dismantled, and the wind outside was blowing so strongly that it felt like our tent would be ripped away before the Sherpas could dismantle it! As I stepped out into the blinding sunlight, I felt like I was in the arctic because the winds and cold were "biting to the bone." My down clothing would not be coming off in this weather.

The trip from Camp 4 to the Geneva Spur was quite perilous: the blowing snow had covered the trail, and with no fixed ropes on this section it was more disconcerting. Once over the spur, the trail was a steady descent that crossed the Yellow Band and then progressed down to Camp 3. At Camp 3 all of the tents had been dismantled because all of the teams had already left the mountain. We were actually the last team to summit, and I had been the last person to stand on top of the world; no one else came up the mountain as I descended. From Camp 3, we again faced serious descent challenges, and the extreme angle of the Lhotse Face slowed my descent again to a snail's pace.

MyEverest Blog

Keep that big v8 "motor" of yours topped up with high octane "fuel," select low gear and you'll be at camp 3 before you can say "Jeff Gordon." All the best, good health, good climbing!!!—ken.nz

My legs now felt like rubber, and again I fell a few times, yet these falls were more terrifying than those on the summit because the extreme angle was much more frightening. It took longer to recover from each fall, and my confidence was slowly leaving me. I did not know whether I had what was needed to make it off the Lhotse Face. On the final pitch, with the end in sight, I again fell, for the last time! This time I slid for a while, but as with all the other falls, was eventually safe. I rested for quite a long time before I managed to get to the bottom of the Lhotse Face. Then I collapsed. I have never been so exhausted in all my life! I still had another 1-1/2 hours on a gradual slope to Camp 2, was being "fried" by the intense sun, had no fluids left, and was very, very weak! I made it to Camp 2 "on fumes" and was treated to a fantastic meal and enough fluids to sink a ship. It was great to be almost down the mountain, but I could not relax until tomorrow when I got to Base Camp.

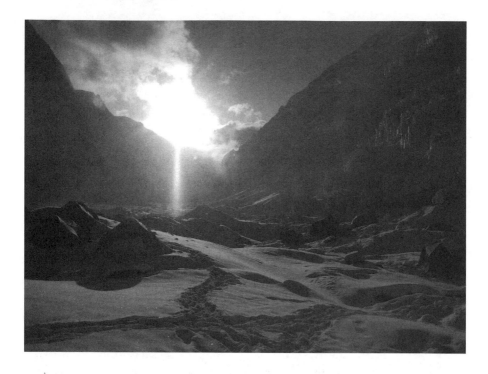

MyEverest Blog

Good luck and safe climbing. In the bicycling world we always say "keep the rubber side down and the shiny side up." Whatever is the mountaineering equivalent (keep your feet on the ground and your head in the sky?), have a great time.—JQ

Life-Changing Risk

Sleep was deep and intense that night at Camp 2; however, the calm was punctuated by the roar of frequent avalanches all night long! The topography had changed drastically since we were here 4 days ago: almost all the snow in camp had melted, and there were now small streams on the trail because the seasonal changes brought warmer temperatures. With that in mind, we departed Camp 2 very early in the morning. We wanted to get through the Khumbu, our last and final trip, as fast as we could to avoid any potential problems. However, an additional challenge would confront us prior to departure: all of our excess gear, which had been stowed at Camp 2, now had to be carried down the mountain by its owners. This extra weight greatly added to the burden of the trip and turned an already exhausting ordeal into an overwhelming challenge. Tired legs, exhausted and dehydrated bodies, and minds that were still cloudy from the effects of the previous day's altitude and time in the death zone were accidents waiting to happen. Undaunted, we forged forward and after a little over an hour we were at Camp 1. While all the others took a quick break, I continued onward: I had found my second wind, was in marathon mode, and did not want to slow until I reached the bottom.

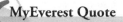

MyEverest Quote

"It is not the mountain we conquer but ourselves."—Sir Edmund Hillary

As with Camp 2, a lot of the topography here was changing in the Khumbu, and the route down had changed quite significantly since we last were here. Effortless ladder crossings weeks ago now required crawling across on hands and knees. Snow bridges across gaping crevasses had started to open, and all along the trail there were huge gaps that required circumnavigation to reach the other side. At the lower part of the Khumbu, there were now small streams to navigate because of melted icefall, and it became very challenging to follow the trail because the streams now carved new routes into the glacier. This was quite disconcerting, and I was very worried about the solidity of the taller ice structures towering over us on the trail. As I descended, my thoughts were focused on my wife and family, and I silently sent prayers of thanks for making it this far. But I still could not relax, not until I made it to Base Camp.

MyEverest Blog

What a fantastic, insane, amazing, inspirational feat you and the team have done. It is such a team but individual effort. It was so amazing to hear your voice from the top of the world. It has been an exciting journey to have been able to follow you all the way to the top and back. I am so glad & relieved that you are all safe and intact. Top of the world to you!—LS

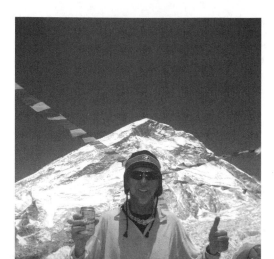

Living the Dream

In record time, and without incident, I slowly walked into Base Camp ahead of our team. On entry to the fringe of camp, I was greeted by a welcoming party of well-wishers who were waiting for one of their team members whom I had met and passed about 30 minutes earlier. After giving them an update on their friend, and telling them that I had just completed my summit of **Mt. Everest**, I started to walk away. However, my walk was halted by the screaming and cheering of this crowd of about 30 strangers as they celebrated my completion of a 7-year odyssey. How fitting to have my journey end with a group of strangers who had now become friends. On all of my climbs around the world, I had always met and climbed with strangers, who eventually became friends, and then family. The camaraderie of climbers is epic because we literally die to save each other! What a relief, what a relief, what a relief! I celebrated my arrival with the Base Camp team, and as my climbing team members arrived we celebrated some more. For all, it was a celebration of survival, and life, because we had made it to the top and down safely.

> ## MyEverest Quote
>
> "You cannot be a good mountaineer, however great your ability, unless you are cheerful and have the spirit of comradeship. Friends are as important as achievement. Another is that teamwork is the one key to success and that selfishness only makes a man small. Still another is that no man, on a mountain or elsewhere, gets more out of anything than he puts into it."—Tenzing Norgay

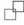

Table 5-1   Attitude Checklist

Review the following list to see how you can change your attitude.

Attitude Adjustment	Yes	No
Self		
• Have a positive attitude		
• Am happy with my physical looks		
• Am happy with my physical health		
• Am able to change attitude when: – Needed – Requested		
• Am reliable and honest		
Relationships		
• Am considerate of others' feelings		
• Constantly compliment people		
• Am courteous to others		
• Respect opinions and beliefs of others		
• In the last week I have had a positive attitude toward: – Family – Friends – Coworkers – Significant other		
• Always look for the best in everyone		
• Always find the silver lining		

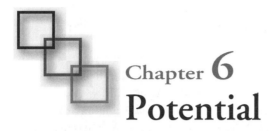

Chapter **6**

Potential

One day a farmer's donkey fell into an abandoned well. The animal cried piteously for hours as the farmer tried to figure out what to do. Finally, he decided the animal was old and the well needed to be covered up anyway; so it just wasn't worth it to him to retrieve the donkey.

He invited all his neighbors to come over and help him. They each grabbed a shovel and began to shovel dirt into the well. Realizing what was happening, the donkey at first cried and wailed horribly. Then, a few shovelfuls later, he quieted down completely.

The farmer peered down into the well, and was astounded by what he saw. With every shovelful of dirt that hit his back, the donkey was doing something amazing. He would shake it off and take a step up on the new layer of dirt. As the farmer's neighbors continued to shovel dirt on top of the animal, he would continue to shake it off and take a step up.

Pretty soon, the donkey stepped up over the edge of the well and trotted off, to the shock and astonishment of the neighbors. Life's going to shovel dirt on you, all kinds of dirt. The trick to getting out of the well is not to let it bury you, but to shake it off and take a step up. Each of our troubles is a stepping stone. We can get out of the deepest wells just by not stopping, never giving up! Shake it off and take a step up!

—ANONYMOUS

What is potential, and how do we know if we have it? If we do have it, how is it measured? Why do people say it is important to use our potential, and how do we tap into that potential? According to *Merriam-Webster's Collegiate Dictionary*, 11th edition, the word *potential* is derived from the Latin word for *power* and can be used as a verb phrase in "expressing possibility, liberty, or power." A common interpretation of potential is that it refers to the possibility, likelihood, or sometimes expectation that a person has the capacity to do better in his or her life. But how is this determined, and what are the measures? Historically, potential was measured using a variety of testing methods, including the intelligent quotient (IQ) test. The prevailing thought in the early 1900s was that the IQ test could measure a child's intelligence, which supposedly would be an indication of his or her potential in life. There has been much consternation about this approach: both teachers and parents feel strongly that IQ results can falsely label children as being intelligent, or not, and can set them up to fail. In today's scholastic setting, we make use of quantitative indicators such as grades, test scores, and grade point average (GPA) to measure potential, but we fail to take into account a person's drive to succeed against more challenging odds in life, as well as their true strengths.

Raising Your Standards

Another challenge facing us in schools is our use of traditional testing methods, such as exams, writing assignments, and quizzes, and how this knowledge is applied in the real world, or, in the case of nursing, the clinical setting. Does a student who excels in the didactic portion of a course but not in the application process in the clinical setting show less potential than a student who excels in the clinical setting but not in the classroom setting? When students progress from school to work, they are then exposed to further methods for measuring potential, including scales of intelligence, problem-solving ability (cognitive ability), motivation, personality, and educational or developmental needs to succeed.

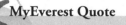

MyEverest Quote

"Patience and perseverance have a magical effect before which difficulties disappear and obstacles vanish."
—John Quincy Adams

My Travels Through Life

While Dad wrestled with managing two jobs and family life, I developed as a kid and started to explore my own little world. Directly across the street from my house was a rail line that fed into a railroad yard not half a mile distant. I can remember hopping those trains as they slowly crawled through the city making their way to parts of the country unknown to me. I can vividly recall wondering what it was like to be a hobo and to travel for free on these trains with no worries in the world except for your next meal and a place to sleep. I saw those hobos occasionally and always respected them for their worldliness; after all, what was more important than exploration and seeing sights unseen? Hopping those trains was no easy feat, because there was risk of capture by the train police. I am sure that there was probably some imminent danger associated with falling off a train and getting crushed or killed, but I was invincible as a kid, and that factor never even crossed my mind! I remember climbing aboard the open boxcars and riding them from the train yard to my house. The half-mile distance seemed so far, yet so near, because here I would have to exit with a well-planned roll in the ditch. My heart would always fill with anticipation when the chiming crosswalk bells close to my house signaled that it was nearing time to jump.

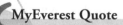

MyEverest Quote

"I hoped that the trip would be the best of all journeys; a journey into ourselves."—Shirley MacLaine

In that short trip, I allowed my mind to wander many times to faraway places with names I had only heard, but wanted to see. My initial dream stops were Toronto and Montreal: their hockey teams were Canada's pride, and I was a die-hard fan. Once past those areas, I imagined stopping in either New York or Chicago, because their hockey teams were represented on the "foosball-type game" that Dad would give us each Christmas. My world at that time existed only in terms of hockey cities, because in Canada in the mid-1950s hockey ruled! After being given those games for Christmas, my brothers and I would draw straws to see who would get to be the American team. We all were very patriotic, and no one wanted to be the Americans. Quite ironic, now that I have spent over half of my life in that country that none of my brothers, nor I, wanted to represent in the hockey game. I think that I got the short straw quite often, which must have been a sign.

MyEverest Blog

"Testing one's limits may create a risk factor but it is the only way to find out what you are truly capable of."—MC

The Moment

Not far away from the house was the Ottawa River, another magical playground. Here the shores were lined with the carcasses of huge trees that were cut down upriver and floated to a lumber mill in Hull, Quebec, for production as building material. These logs provided an opportunity for hours of fun as I grew adept at stealthily managing my way across the tops of the logs without being dunked in the river. To fall meant that the logs would roll overhead and trap you underwater; the pure weight of these dead trees were massive even in the water, where they floated easily. It was here that I learned to hold my breath for extended periods of time and calmly navigate my way under the logs that had thrown me off. I later learned to resist the logs' futile attempts to throw me in the water and always maintained my calm. I felt serenity underwater, no doubt linked to my horoscope sign (Pisces), and I found peace in the cold depths. It was here, too, that I saved a life for the first time, another sign of things to come. A new friend had fallen off the logs and was trapped beneath them, but could not swim. I found him easily underwater as he tried futilely to claw his way out of the shadows above him. I remember the panic in his eyes: he knew he could not breathe and did not know where to go. I took him by the hand and pulled him to daylight and life. He survived, but it wasn't the last time that I would attempt to save his life.

MyEverest Blog

"It is the driving force of the human spirit that propels us to do great things."—MC

If It Works Once, Try It Again

When winter came and the river had frozen, we retreated indoors to the warmth and security of heated pools as a respite from the cold weather. It was here that my friend once again found himself in a precarious position—drowning in a pool. I recalled from our earlier situation that he was a weak swimmer, and in fact I don't think I had ever seen him swim. I knew that he could sink like a rock, because our first encounter had been at the bottom of the Ottawa River beneath a logjam. I quickly swam over to grab him from the deep end of the pool and guide him to safety as I had done before; however, the unexpected occurred, and I found myself being pushed underwater as he used my shoulders to keep his head above water. I tried to struggle and fight him off, but a drowning person's strength and panic are overwhelming. I remember a flurry of activity as his feet kicked my face and shoulders, which pushed me deeper and deeper into the depths of the pool. And then there was calm, and time stood still. I remember a deep, deep black, yet the pool was well lit. It was peaceful, but alarming. Why was I seeing pictures of my family, and why couldn't I speak? And then I looked up into the eyes of a stranger who had his mouth on mine, and suddenly I was coughing and gagging as water spewed from my mouth and lungs. I was lying along the side of the pool, and my chest was burning and my ribs were sore. The lifeguard who pulled me from the bottom of the pool had saved my life by doing CPR. Sitting across from me was the friend I had saved, wrapped in a towel and looking quite shocked, but no worse for the wear. At least we were both alive. Still, today I feel serenity in the water, and a peaceful calm overcomes me whenever I dive. However, swimming has always been a challenge.

Teachers ... Who Needs Them?

MyEverest Quote

"On the mountains of truth you can never climb in vain; either you will reach a point higher up today, or you will be training your powers so that you will be able to climb higher tomorrow."—Friedrich Nietzsche

I feel that I have come full circle in life, because I have become what I fought against all my life: a teacher. As I reflect on my career as a student, I have to apologize to all the teachers who ever had me in their class, because I seemed to always go out of my way to make their life just a little more challenging than it really had to be. Don't get me wrong: I was not a bad student, but more of a problem student in that I was always doing something to "get on their nerves." For some reason, I could not accept the status quo and questioned everything and everyone. I am sure that some of this stemmed from my desire to be noticed, because I did act the fool in class and was always competing to be the class clown. I was an ugly duckling as a child, the firstborn of eight boys and one girl, and terribly insecure. My attempts to be noticed helped alleviate that insecurity, but I had to go to extremes to do so. These extremes caught the attention of both students and teachers, but usually the teachers were left with the lasting impression because they were the ones who had to "set me straight." I can remember many times having to write on the chalkboard that I would not repeat the behavior that got me in trouble. And here I am, 40 years later, again writing on that chalkboard, but this time I'm not in trouble.

MyEverest Quote

"Greatness lies not in being strong, but in the right use of strength."—Henry Ward Beecher

When I think of those who made a difference in my life, I have to say that teachers were the most dominant. All of them had a clear vision of where we were as students and where we needed to be; it was just very problematic for them to have us share in this vision. My primary school, St. Mary's, was located in the shadows of the church spires, and our playground was the parking lot for people attending Mass. My teachers were the Sisters of St. Joseph, and their convent was located at the other end of the parking lot. As a young student, I feared these ladies, because their stern, hardened ways were difficult for me to accept. Yet I smiled when seeing them in their long, dark, flowing robes with heads covered in white, because they reminded me of penguins. I liked to laugh, play jokes, and be the center of attention, but they thought they should have center stage in class. Needless to say, we had many "come to Jesus" meetings, and I became a collective project for all of the nuns. They decided to keep a close watch on me, so they worked it out with my mom to have me clean the local convent as a part-time job after school. Here I got to see the nuns without their habits and saw that they were real people after all.

As a result of their concentrated efforts, I became an altar boy and assisted the priests when conducting Mass. The view of the church from the altar is very humbling, because you get to see the entire congregation in prayer. I progressed from altar boy to doing the readings from the pulpit, and this was my first attempt at public speaking before large groups of people. I can always remember grabbing the edges of the pulpit so tightly that I felt I left indentations in the wood, because my initial nervousness was so great. Thirty years later I reflected on this church experience when I stood before thousands of perioperative nurses to give a speech that resulted in my position on the national board of directors for the Association of periOperative Registered Nurses (AORN). On that day, I again dug my fingers deep into the podium but soon relaxed as the initial stage fright passed and the wave of nausea soon after.

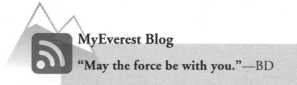

MyEverest Blog

"May the force be with you."—BD

Another of my primary school teachers who left an indelible mark on my being was a red-headed Irishman. His whimsical tales of travel abroad excited me to no end. Here was a man who had traveled the world and shared those stories with us in class. I was spellbound most of the time, and I am sure a seed was planted by him, because my desire for travel and adventure had just begun. From primary school, I transitioned to a boys' Catholic high school in a city 30 miles away from my family. Mom and Dad felt that I needed a more strictly regimented high school experience, because the hard work of the nuns and other teachers in primary school had not given the desired result of a model student.

Realizing the Possibilities

Additionally, it seemed that Mom was hoping that as the eldest male I would become a priest, and this exposure to priests might help straighten out my wayward ways and help me to concentrate on her expectations of what lay ahead in my future. Unfortunately, she had not shared her vision with me, and I felt I was being banished to another world because this was not where I wanted to be. I missed my grade-school friends who were attending high school in my hometown. I did, however, make the best of a bad situation and developed an appreciation for Latin, learned the skills required to live away from home, and developed a closer bond to my grandmother, with whom I lived. The teachers there were very stern priests, and I am sure it helped give me better direction in life, yet I was still confused about what I wanted to do "when I grew up." I do remember that the two years of private Catholic high school reinforced that I did not want to be priest, although I did discover an affinity for wanting to help people.

My next transition was from the city high school to the country high school, where I was able to reunite with my grade-school friends. There I had the opportunity to participate in sports despite the family doctor's stern warning of the potential onset of asthma attacks. I excelled in football and track but warmed the bench for basketball. The camaraderie of team sports has been everlasting because the friends I made then are friends for life, and lessons we learned on the football field have helped me put life in perspective. Together we can achieve more.

MyEverest Blog

"Allow things to fall into place by setting up the groundwork for things to fall into."—MC

It was there in that tiny country high school that my life would forever be changed by a few teachers who were just doing their jobs. My history teacher painted a swath of excitement for me when he took a dry topic and made it come alive. Wars, conquests, and political strife all sprang to life for me as he made the years and places seem so close. Building on this teacher's information was my geography teacher, who opened the world to me by describing lands and people in faraway places that I had no idea existed. I am certain that this class helped the seed that had been planted in primary school to grow and flourish as a flower, because the tales of languages and cultures excited me to no end. In fact, it was during high school that I was able to take my first trip abroad. This high school trip to Greece was a class excursion, so I was able to share my excitement with my best friends. I was hooked, line and sinker, because it was everything that I dreamed it would be, and then some! Wow, to walk among Greek ruins, to see the birthplace of the Olympics, and to eat ethnic food and listen to the language of another culture was simply overwhelming. Looking back now, over 34 years later, I can see that it was this trip and the history/geography classes that confirmed for me my dreams of travel and adventure. It was exciting, and I loved it!

My trip to Greece was 57 countries ago, and my wife Carol and I have shared this common love of travel and adventure for the past 24 years. This love has also taken me down paths that I would never have imagined, because I have been able to combine my nursing experience and travel to better the lives of those in other countries. For the past 14 years, I have been involved in the organization Partners of the Americas, which has allowed me to send multiple shipments of medical supplies to Colombia in South America. Additionally, a yearlong trip through Latin America helped me decide that my doctoral dissertation would focus on the barriers that Hispanics face when trying to access health care.

MyEverest Blog

"It is a spark in the imagination that will ignite your creativity and set you on fire."—MC

The Road Not Taken

Robert Frost noted in the "The Road Not Taken" that taking the same path as everyone else will get you only average or mediocre results. To be unique, to contribute something new, you need to take a different course—your own. It is far easier to follow the beaten path and enjoy the security of conformity. The steps to realizing your own potential begin first with a clear definition of your goals and objectives. Without a clear vision, your ability to achieve goals can be drastically limited. The next step is to create a plan, because most goals don't happen by accident. The plan must be realistic and viable, meaning that if followed, it has a reasonable likelihood of success. Dreaming of climbing **Mt. Everest** is one thing, but actually getting out of a plane in Kathmandu, Nepal, with your gear is another.

MyEverest Blog

You're doing it my man!! All your hard work and dedication is going to pay off!! This is where you have to dig down deep! Just like any sport ... you have to work through the pain. One step at a time ... But just be smart about it! Make sure you give yourself enough time to turn around if you have to! Really pushing for you!! This is amazing stuff!!—Anonymous

The next step involves your ability to overcome obstacles, problems, challenges, and unforeseeable setbacks. These will happen, and the key is to be prepared both mentally and physically. Perseverance is the next step and requires the greatest investment in time and resources. Having a commitment to persevere, especially when faced with obstacles, is a key differentiator between achievement and failure. If I had listened to all the people who had many reasons why I should not climb **Mt. Everest**, I never would have gotten there. Involvement of others—family, friends, and teammates—is the next step and a very critical one because rarely do people become successful alone. Individual and team goals are greatly impacted by your abilities to delegate, ask for assistance, and solicit support from friends, mentors, and others who have experience in the area of your pursuit. Teamwork is what got me to the top of all my summits. The final step to realizing your potential is the knowledge that it will require building upon partial successes. Most major personal achievements are the culmination of many little ones, with each of the smaller achievements providing important steps that lead to success. It was a culmination of training on smaller mountains that prepared me to take on the bigger challenges of the 7 Summits of the World.

MyEverest Blog

There was a thought for the day in our Sunday epistle today that made me think of you when I read it. I wanted to share it with you: "We must learn to acknowledge that the creation is full of mystery; we will never entirely understand it. We must abandon arrogance and stand in awe. We must recover the sense of the majesty of creation and the ability to be worshipful in its presence. For I do not doubt that it is only on the condition of humility and reverence before the world that our species will be able to remain in it."—CT

My Journey in Nursing

We all became nurses for different reasons. Many have had family members who were nurses or in the medical profession; others had experiences with relatives who were sick and were lovingly cared for by nurses; still others were influenced by a family member or friend who told them that they had a comforting disposition that would become a nurse. My entry into this profession was quite different: a high school guidance counselor recommended that I pursue nursing. I was the oldest of nine children and lived on a farm in rural Ontario. As a high school student I had no idea what I wanted to do ... but I hadn't even considered nursing. I had never been admitted to a hospital, and my only interactions with those in the medical field had been through visits to the doctor's office and the emergency room for treatment of asthma. Additionally, I had no idea whether I had any of the essential qualities necessary to be a nurse. I suspected that my mom would have been happy if I had become a Catholic priest; however, that meant church every Saturday night and Sunday morning and I didn't think that I could commit to that hectic schedule! My dad would have been happy if I had taken over the farm because we had a lot of cattle and much potential for growth, but I had asthma and lots of allergies that caused me all kinds of problems when working in the barn. So, when this guidance counselor suggested nursing, it came as kind of a shock.

Who Do We Think We Are?

I will never forget the day that I met with my guidance counselor to go over her top three recommendations for careers. Her first recommendation was childcare worker—nope, wouldn't work because I did not have a strong affection for kids. Her second recommendation was prison guard—nope, wouldn't work because I have always had nightmares of being imprisoned. And her third and final recommendation was the most disturbing: nursing. I felt hurt, upset, and disappointed.

Why did she suggest a nursing career to me? I thought that she liked me. Had I done something wrong to have her want to steer me down a path less traveled by men? Were there questions of my masculinity that I did not know how to answer? Why nursing? At that point in my life, I had little interaction with health care, and no one in our family worked in medicine. What did she see in me that I did not see in myself? This was very troublesome, because I respected Mrs. Lamb and did not expect to hear this from her. I felt like the wind had been knocked out of me as it did during a hard hit in football. I needed to get air. I jumped up to rush out, and I barely heard her directions to attend a meeting the following week when a college representative would visit our school to discuss nursing.

During the week following that meeting, I kept to myself and never uttered a word to friends or family of my meeting with Mrs. Lamb. Who was she anyway, and what did she know? I wanted to be a reporter and travel the world writing articles on people and places and experience the smell and taste of foreign foods. I wanted to speak in other languages and live in straw huts. I wanted to ride trains, float down rivers in rafts, and discover villages of people deep in thick jungles. How could I do that as a nurse, and why would I want to be a nurse? Yes, I had a strong Catholic upbringing and was a very sensitive person, but I had no idea about medicine and very little exposure to health care. Mom had suffered from varicose veins all her life and I had seen them rupture on occasion, only to have Dad elevate her leg and place a pail beneath the bleeding leg to make certain that it did not mess up the floor. Perhaps a nurse in the family was needed? I did recall my brother's emergency with amputated fingers and finding those macerated digits in the field. The only other medical experiences I had at that time were associated with farm life: the birth and caring of animals as well as the slaughter of those same animals for food on our table.

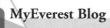

MyEverest Blog

"I believe our dreams do not define us … they drive us. Rather, it's the moments and how we receive them that truly define us …"—L

I went that next week and attended the meeting on nursing—and guess what, I was the only guy in the room! But everything that representative said was pretty cool, and I actually left with a different impression of nursing. I remembered that this college recruiter said it was a caring profession and that you would help the sick to become better and enable them to live a longer life. Wow, an opportunity to help people to live longer: this must be a miracle profession! I thought that only doctors had that power. The recruiter also said that the nurses received very good wages, and as a nurse you could work anywhere in the world. Hey, maybe this was a way that I could feed my hunger for travel and adventure. I do remember going home that day and telling my parents that I was considering becoming a nurse. Mom was extremely happy because she felt it was in line with her priesthood wishes (sacrifice, poverty, and servitude); however, Dad was not too happy. He basically said that no damn son of his would ever become a nurse and stormed out of the room. It took me a little longer to tell my high school friends because even though it sounded exciting to me, I felt I was going to have a hard time getting them to feel the excitement. After all, most of my friends were seeking careers as architects, lawyers, doctors, and accountants. How could I compete with those professions as a nurse?

MyEverest Blog

"The reward is not in the acknowledgment of helping a fellow human being; it is in the act itself."—MC

The First Step

However, the nursing program was not what I thought it would be, and I faced challenge after challenge of trying to comprehend the materials, learn medical terminology, and make sense of everything. This was my second time away from home, I was still unsure of my potential, and I probably partied a little too much, which took me away from my studies. Somehow I mustered the courage to approach one of my clinical instructors and confessed that I was fearful of failing the program. I told my instructor that I felt I had made an enormous mistake, because I did not feel that I was meant to be a nurse. Up until that point, I had always taken the easiest patient assignments, those that had one or two medications and were hopefully being discharged soon. Additionally, I was always overwhelmed by the course content, and I constantly found myself reading, writing, and preparing for class while other students were enjoying the extracurricular activities of college life. I'll never forget that day with my instructor, because she took the time to talk with me and basically said that I was not challenging myself enough. She also said that she knew I had the potential to do well, but was not applying myself as I should. My instructor wanted me to excel and decided to challenge me by assigning me the most complicated patients. What an idiot I was! This is not what I wanted. This was way too overwhelming, and I was not sure whether I would sink or swim—but guess what: I survived and was a better person for it.

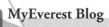

MyEverest Blog

Today I went to a friend's house for her daughter's high school graduation. Her daughter is a CNA and enrolled in a potential nursing program—but, her daughter told me tonight she doesn't know if she wants to be a nurse, because her observation is that all nurses do is paperwork! So now (needless to say) I am on a bandwagon to let her know how exciting nursing is and the clinical judgments that are involved are invigorating and, yes, we need to document things for continuity in care—but the profession of nursing is not just about paperwork. This is the second time I have heard this in a week. Nurses are not just secretaries taking dictation about the status quo (not that there is anything wrong with secretaries, but that is not what nursing is about)—we are shaping the full picture of what is happening from several different inputs. We are the ones that make it all come together and everything talk to each other. We are the GLUE—it makes a difference to have a patient advocate who puts two and two together. So—I need some testimonies from other nurses so I can share them with my friend's daughter—who cared for her dad who died of cancer about 2 years ago. She went into CNA (Certified Nursing Aide) work so she could be hands-on with patients out of the passion for caring for her dad. I am afraid her vision of nursing is that we are not close at hand to the patients. But, I am passionate in believing—we are the ones that bridge the gap—no matter if we work in administration, academics, clinical educators, or in direct patient care.

I plan to tell her about your journey and your Summit scholarship. You may be an extreme example of passion for nursing—but there are many of us who really understand that nursing is something that is different than other professions. There is so much opportunity; so many different pathways in nursing that can be pursued to make a difference in helping people pursue a pathway to wellness. Some of us have 6 to 10 years of education—so I have heard that "you may as well be an MD.." But nursing is different than the medical philosophy! It is its own profession and philosophy and it helps to balance the health care environment with a different take on patient advocacy.—BD

Defining Moments in Life

What are the moments in life that define us? Well, I believe that those moments are right now as we struggle in nursing to prove our value. Nurses have topped Gallup's Honesty and Ethics ranking poll every year but one since they were added to the list in 1999. The exception occurred in 2001 when nurses were bumped off that lofty perch by firefighters shortly after the September 11 terrorist attacks. Each moment that we live helps us to define our being and our potential, and that potential as nurses is to be leaders. As leaders in health care, we make things better for our patients, as well as ourselves; our daily contributions to positive patient outcomes are a reflection on our profession. As patient advocates, we make a difference in our healthcare organizations by working to improve safety at both the individual and organizational levels and do so through our participation on committees, boards, and task forces. As leaders in this volatile healthcare environment, we need to be approachable, accepting, accountable, and most importantly, adaptable.

Our staff members need to be comfortable in approaching us with suggestions and/ or concerns, and when they do, we need to be accepting of these calls for help. We have to be able to acknowledge that change is challenging and takes time, and that it is unrealistic to think that all will see where we want to go at the same time. As leaders we need to be accountable for our actions and admit to our shortcomings. To do so enables our staff members to see that we, too, are human and make mistakes. Adaptability is probably the most valuable component of leadership because it is truly an art and not learned easily. Change is constant in health care; to keep ahead, we must adapt, or else we will quickly fall behind. To function effectively as leaders, we must have a wide range of skills, techniques, and strategies at our disposal, including planning, communication skills, organization, and an awareness of the wider environment in which the team operates.

My Climbs on the Mountains

> ## MyEverest Quote
>
> **"It is better to wear out one's shoes than one's sheets."**—Genoese Proverb

Potential to climb at altitude and in bitterly cold weather is a great unknown, and getting to the top of a mountain is our biggest challenge. As climbers, we are unsure of how we will perform at altitude, because there is always a risk of suffering from a variety of ailments, including HACE, HAPE, dehydration, and hypothermia. To avoid these potential scenarios, we need to make sure that we always have a little extra energy left in us, should an emergency happen, and we need to know how deep those reserves are. Hydration on climbs is vital because the higher altitudes and thinner air can dehydrate a climber very quickly. Rapidly changing temperatures and poor clothing choices can easily contribute to hypothermia. A combination of all the above can occur, to various degrees, which can greatly hinder or cripple a climber's attempt to summit.

However, next to climbing the mountains, some of the most complicating challenges, and paradoxically, exciting events, were simply getting to and from the mountains. Each mountain in its own way was an "Indiana Jones"-type adventure, because travel, accommodations, language, locals, customs, and money were problematic, confusing, and sometimes a bigger obstacle to overcome than the mountains themselves. Three of the 7 Summits of the World stand out in my mind as very problematic to access: **Mt. Vinson** in Antarctica, **Mt. Elbrus** in Russia, and **Carstensz Pyramid** in Indonesia.

MyEverest Blog

"However great your intentions may be, they will remain intentions until you act upon them."—MC

Small Steps to Great Success

On **Mt. Vinson** in Antarctica, my sixth of the 7 Summits of the World, I faced my biggest access challenge, because this area of the world is very, very remote. Located in the middle of Antarctica, this was to be a formidable climb and my testing grounds for the most brutal weather in the world; nighttime temperatures often reach –40. Access to the continent itself proved very problematic because a Russian Ilyushin cargo jet was the only means of transportation, and weather was the determining factor for the flight schedule. After days of waiting in Punta Arenas, Chile, at the very tip of South America, we received word that the weather was favorable and we hastened off to the local airport in preparation for our 6-hour flight. Our seats for the flight were located in the cargo bay of the plane, and our fellow passengers were adventurers from all over the world. Our gear and supplies for the base in Antarctica were strapped down tightly across the floor of the cargo area where we tried to sleep, despite the loud roar of the plane's engines. Our runway on arrival to the continent was deep blue ice, and with no crosswind to challenge our landing, we were able to land safely on a runway that could have been suitable for skating. The desolation of snow and ice spread as far as the eye could see and was only slightly interrupted by some makeshift, temporary huts and tents; evidently survival here was possible only for a short while. A crew of New Zealanders and Canadians maintain this base at Patriot Hills for only 1 to 2 months and then abandon it when the extreme weather rules the barren landscape.

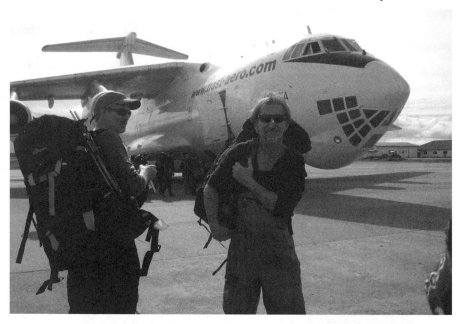

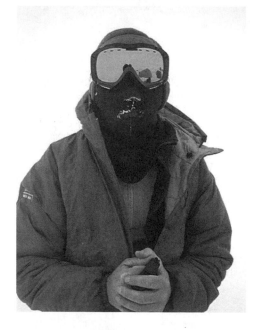

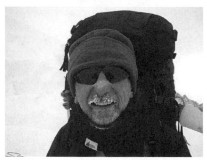

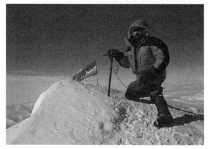

We spent our first night in tents on this windswept landscape, and the next morning we were flown in Twin Otters to **Mt. Vinson** Base Camp. The climb and conditions were very memorable, but it was the getting in and out that was the most exciting. After a successful summit, we eventually made our way back to **Mt. Vinson** Base Camp, where we were most fortunate to be airlifted back to Patriot Hills later that night, just in time to celebrate Christmas. It was December 25, 2006, and we stepped off the Twin Otter planes in Patriot Hills to see Santa Claus, in his red-robed splendor, having a relaxing drink at an outdoor bar, which was carved out of ice with chainsaws. Santa, in reality, was a member of a British climbing team that had encountered a bad storm, and all were suffering from frostbite. The Santa outfit put all of us in a great

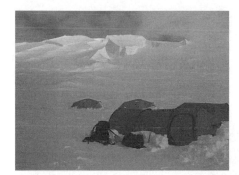 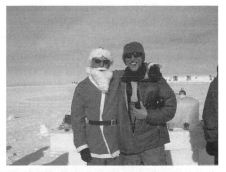

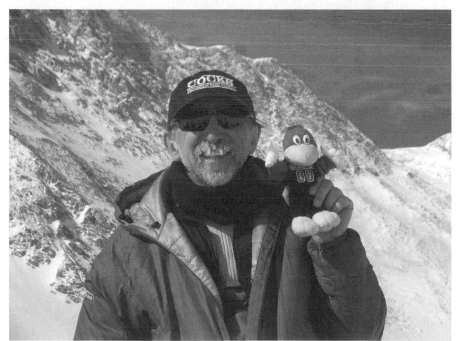

celebratory mood, despite the −20 degree temperatures. As luck would have it, we were able to fly out that night on the Ilyushin cargo jet that had just arrived to drop off fuel. We found out the following day that after our flight landed in Chile, the jet was disabled and was unable to return to Antarctica for another week due to repairs.

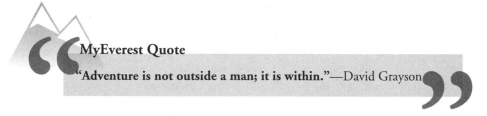

MyEverest Quote

"Adventure is not outside a man; it is within."—David Grayson

Access to **Mt. Elbrus** in Russia, my fourth of the 7 Summits of the World, became problematic when I flew from Moscow to Mineralnye Vody in southern Russia. On arrival at this airport, my team of climbers—composed of South Africans, Danes, Norwegians, and I—were met by a tour guide who was to drive us by van to the Baksan Valley, at the base of **Mt. Elbrus**, located in the Caucasus mountain range. Our departure from the airport was initially delayed by two of the climbers who were arrested by Russian guards for urinating along the side of a building. In their urgency to relieve themselves, they failed to read the sign, written in Russian, which spelled out that this

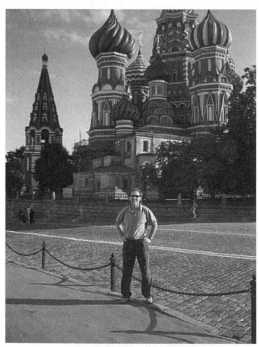

action would be punished by penalties and fines. Hours later, minus hundreds of dollars, our team members walked out of captivity and into our waiting van.

However, our brush with the authorities was not over yet. There happened to be another problem, one that affected me: my name was not listed on the travel itinerary. Our guide was very noticeably nervous as he explained that it was against the law for me to leave the airport if not on the list. I calmly explained that I had flown halfway across the world to climb a mountain and was not going to let a typographical error ruin my trip. At this point, the South African climbers decided to take control

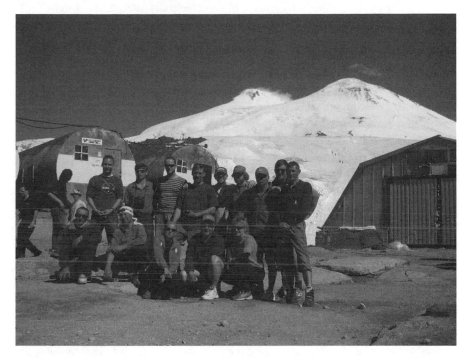

and suggested that I hide in the back of the van, where they would cover me with all of the luggage and backpacks. It sounded like a good plan to me, so I took my place at the back of the van, covered with luggage, and we slowly began to exit the airport. Just as quickly as we had started to move, we began to slow and came to a stop. What was happening? Why had we stopped? Why wasn't anyone saying anything?

And then I heard him, the airport military guard. In broken English, he was asking for everyone's passport. As I slowly moved my head under the pile of bags, I could barely catch a glimpse of this machine gun-toting, stern-faced, huge

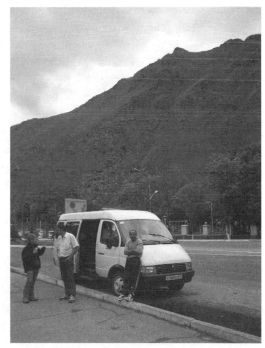

Russian guard. I could hear my heart pounding and hoped that it would not give me away. I tried to wish my heart to stop pounding so loud, but it only raced faster. I felt at one moment that the guard's eyes locked on mine as he cast a glance toward the mess of backpacks and bags that were covering me, and it was at that moment that my heart froze. His eyes were cold and emotionless, and there were no smile creases on his face—not a good sign! In a flash, I pictured him pulling the bags off me, being carted in handcuffs to a Russian prison, and being jailed without recourse for release. In that same instant, I pictured my wife, friends, family, and colleagues, all flashing before my eyes as if in a slide show of a trip. In what seemed like an eternity, his glance moved away from the bags and I heard the first beat of my heart, loud. The guard told the driver that he would be doing a passport check against the trip itinerary to make sure that all was correct, and then he was gone. Wow, the driver had been correct! This was serious business, and now made worse because I was stowed away in the back of a van attempting to be smuggled into southern Russia.

The silence was deafening. No one spoke a word, even though they sat within a few feet of where I lay under the packs and bags. As best I could tell, other guards were walking on and off the van to reinforce their presence, control, and no doubt increase our anxiety. Seconds turned to minutes, and minutes to hours. When the first guard returned with passports in hand, 2 hours had passed. I was able to see and hear him arguing with our driver, and my anxiety went up a few more levels when I felt that he was questioning my presence, or lack thereof. The arguing abated when the driver handed the guard a large wad of what I could only imagine was money, at which point the passports were surrendered to the climbers. The sound of the van starting was music to my ears and the forward motion that I had longed for was now happening. But what was going on? Were we truly departing the airport, or being directed to another area for a detailed search of bags and belongings?

After a few minutes of motion and acceleration, I started to feel bags being removed from on top of me, and I looked up to see one of my South African climbers brandishing a bottle of vodka and heard him say the sweetest, but ironically most provocative words, "Welcome to Russia." This welcome was followed by a cheer as all others were finally able to release pent-up anxiety because they, too, had felt the pressure of the inspection and had individually thought of imprisonment for being accomplices. I joined in the celebrations and thanked everyone profusely for their silent support. The driver was still mortified, because he had never done this before, or so we thought. He relayed to us that we would continue to be checked en route to our destination at roadblocks strategically set up along all highways. Sure enough, only a few miles down the road, we saw the distinctive Russian roadblock that was comprised of a small building located in the center of the road, with a swing gate to stop the flow of traffic. Before slowing, I crawled under the bags again and found my hiding place, which sufficed for that inspection, and all others along our 6-hour journey. What a trip, what an adventure, and we had not even started to climb yet!

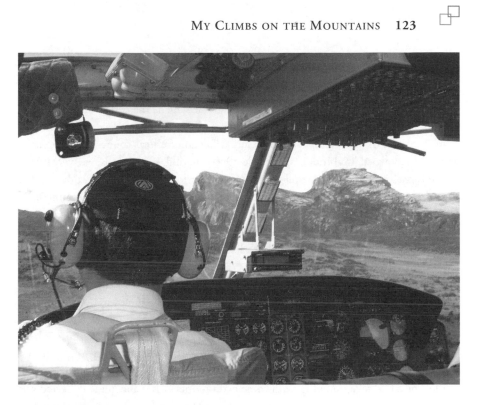

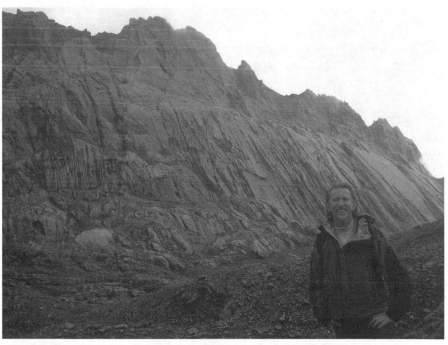

Access to **Carstensz Pyramid** in Indonesia, my fifth of the 7 Summits of the World, was truly an adventure that started a year before I even arrived on the mountain. Due to political unrest, this mountain had been off limits for years and no one had been able to legally climb to the summit. I say "legally" because few made the climb but were arrested and paid hefty fines to be released from prison. Two other climbers and I had been quite persistent in our attempts to climb and unified our efforts to focus our attention on a well-renowned local Indonesian guide. Over a period of 6 months, we were finally able to organize our flights, supplies, and plans. Our local guide had reassured us that this climb would be the first legal one in three years and would open this mountain to the rest of the world, which had been waiting so patiently for the government problems to be resolved. I met my two climbing mates in the Singapore airport and was in awe of their climbing experience because both had done big-wall climbing, which involves climbing extreme vertical rock faces, such as El Capitan in Yosemite National Park, and this was to be last of their 7 Summits of the World. I was in great hands.

However, our bubble of enthusiasm for a well-organized climb was burst on arrival in Manado, on the island of Sulawesi. Our local guide reaffirmed our worst fears: that we did not have government permission to climb the mountain. Why did we have to find this out now after traveling halfway around the world and spending untold thousands of dollars? Our guide had known of this problem before our departures, but felt he could take care of it, with some extra money! After the guide collected our

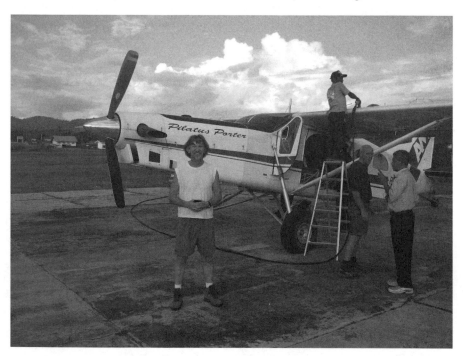

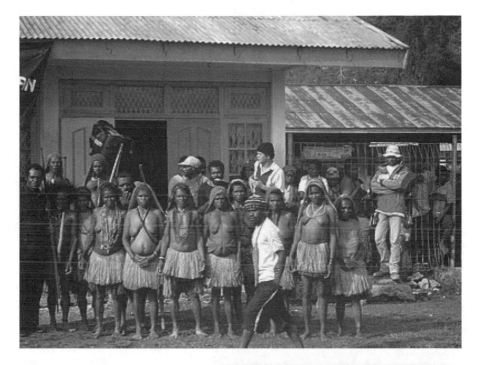

money, we decided that we would move forward with the attempt to climb and possibly along the way we could gain some local support. Our number one priority became the need to physically get to the base of the mountain, in whatever way we could, because we felt if we could get there we could climb and hopefully escape under the radar screen of attention.

Travel to New Guinea required a flight from Manado across the Molucca Sea to the island of Biak for an overnight stay, and then further travel to the coastal town of Nabire, located in Irian Jaya, Indonesia. Because it was high season for locals, and we had no reservations, we had to beg, borrow, and

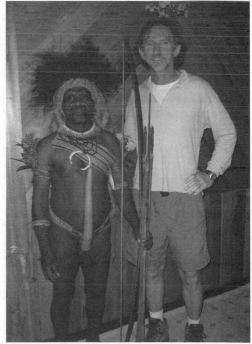

plead to get seats on these small planes. There is no doubt that the extra money that we collected helped give us bargaining power. After we landed in Nabire, we had to fly into the mountains, and it was there that our guide started to make deals with government helicopter pilots as well as local private pilots. After a few days of waiting and visits to military encampments seeking permission to climb, we were fortunate to be able to pay to be "smuggled" up to Enarotali, a mountain village at 5,500 feet elevation. Our transport would be in a plane used for missionary flights. As we all crammed into the plane, the pilot showed his distaste for what he was about to do, despite being paid well for his services: he was initially quite rude and questioned our attempts to climb illegally. The flight up into the mountains was through very rugged terrain, and on approach to the short dirt runway, which was carved into the side of a mountain, we had to make a very drastic descent in order to land safely.

As we exited the plane, I was not prepared for our welcome party: we were surrounded by hundreds of local natives, the Dani people. Most were dressed in very little clothing: the women wore straw skirts and nothing else, and a number of the men wore *kotekas*, which are penis sheaths made of dried gourds. The locals milled about us closely, some touching our hair, and most staring in disbelief. Our pilot informed us that missionaries had been here three years earlier, but since then these people had not seen Westerners. Our accommodations were very basic, and the mountain village very

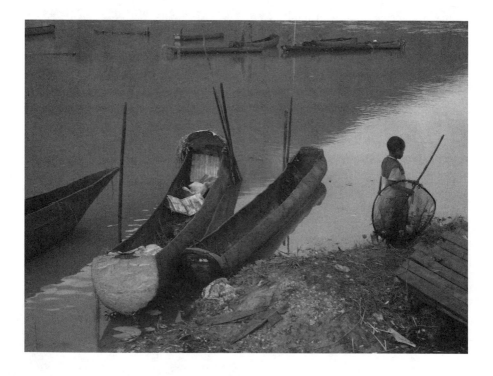

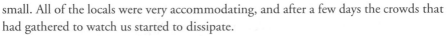

small. All of the locals were very accommodating, and after a few days the crowds that had gathered to watch us started to dissipate.

Before we left this village, I had an opportunity to visit the local hospital/clinic and saw how basic their health care was. There were next to no resources, and people died slow, agonizing deaths from malaria and other tropical diseases. I saw how troubled the nurses were, and on a second trip to the hospital I gave them a box of chocolates that I had bought in the village. Through an interpreter I told them that I knew they were greatly underpaid and overworked, and as a fellow nurse I appreciated all that they did for mankind. On receipt of this gift, two nurses, who were no taller than 4 feet, began to sing and dance around the room. No one had ever given them a present before. For me it was like Christmas—and I enjoyed their gaiety as much as I did when my nieces and nephews opened presents on Christmas Day.

We departed for Base Camp by military helicopter, which was the event of the month because it had quite a long time since a helicopter had dropped out of the sky to land in their village. As we flew into the rugged mountains, I again became concerned: I observed the two pilots charting their course on a tourist map of the island. As a fixed-wing pilot, I know that pilots use detailed navigational maps listing landmarks and elevations to travel between locations, but a tourist map? I brought this to our guide's attention, and he told me that no maps existed, because the area

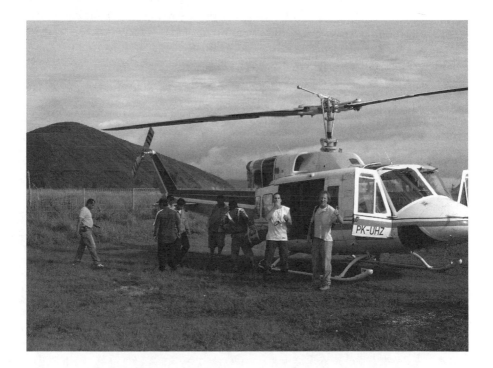

we were headed to was off limits and controlled by the military. Great. What had we gotten ourselves into now? As the pilots flew higher and higher, they started asking our guide for directions, and with the combined efforts of all three, we were able to land at the Zebra Wall, which is the starting place for the trek to high camp. Adjacent to our landing site, at 12,100 feet, was the highest mine in the world, protected by the Indonesian military. It was great news that we would have protection, should we need it, or so I thought!

The climb and summit were memorable, but our departure even more so because the helicopter that dropped us off failed to return as scheduled. Also, we had already run out of food 2 days earlier because our support team failed to arrive due to foul weather. Weakened by the climb, dehydrated, and malnourished, we decided to exit the mountain by crossing the mining area that was heavily patrolled by military. Who would notice four people crossing a vast expanse of upturned rocks and soil, spread across a jagged mountaintop, literally in the middle of nowhere? The Indonesian military would, and did so within minutes of our trespassing. A jeep with four armed guards pulled up to me and used the international sign of pointing a gun barrel first at me, and then waving it in the direction that they wanted me to move. No English needed, just common sense! We were held in the barracks of a military encampment at gunpoint. Our guide, who spoke the language, was taken to a separate facility. Under our breaths we whispered potential scenarios, each of which looked pretty gloomy as the vast number of guards seemed to increase as the day went on. As morning turned into afternoon, the guards started to relax and even fall asleep. One of the guards' semiautomatic rifles was actually resting against my leg while he slept, and his pistol belt was within arm's reach. Through eye movements we climbers communicated with each other, noting that all guards, save for one, were now sleeping. My eyes became as large as saucers when I misinterpreted our plans to be disarming the guards. There was no way that we would survive, but what were their plans?

Shortly afterward they awoke, and it was then that I regretted not disarming our guards because their actions showed that our lives were meaningless to them. All of the guards had cell phones, and most were playing games and/or sending and receiving messages, when suddenly one of the guards became very excited and started to share his phone with all of the others. This was first time that they had shown emotion, and our spirits started to lift because they were now smiling, laughing, hitting, and shoving each other as guys would do when watching something pornographic. We, too, started to smile and laugh among ourselves because we were caught up in the frenzy of the moment, until one of the guards handed us their cell phone to view the video that had been sent to them. Years of caring for patients traumatized by severe injuries sustained in car accidents, explosions, and shootings, as well as years of living on the farm where I helped my Dad slaughter cattle, pigs, and chickens could not prepare me for what I was about to see. On the tiny screen of the cell phone, I saw what appeared to be a captive American soldier with hands bound, reading a prescribed statement, and standing behind him were two hooded men brandishing firearms. As the soldier turned up the volume on the phone, I could now hear the statement being read and looked up to see that all of the guards in the small room were looking at me as if I were going to translate for them. As I looked back at the phone screen, I saw one of the hooded men behind the soldier unsheathe a large sword from his belt, grab the American's head by his hair, and proceeded to slash his throat with large carving motions. Gurgling sounds and a deep cry from the soldier preceded the decapitation, and the soldier's head was now being held by the assailant. I rolled over and started to have dry heaves because I had nothing on my stomach to throw up. The room started spinning, and I felt hot. I had to get out of here. But where could I go? As I looked up between dry heaves, I saw that all of the guards were laughing at me because my response was what they had expected, and then some. I looked at the other climbers for support, and their faces were emotionless.

How could this cruelty happen? And where was this happening? Were we to be next? Was this to be our final climb? As these thoughts and more ran through my mind, suddenly the door to the jail area swung open and there before us stood our local guide, accompanied by what appeared to be an army officer, as indicated by the colorful regalia of bars and ribbons on his uniform. Without saying a word, the officer threw a few boxes at our feet. Dumbfounded by what had just happened, we slowly opened the boxes and were pleasantly surprised to see that they contained chicken and rice. Wow, real food! We had not seen this for almost 5 days and were exhausted from a very physical climb, as well as dehydration, and now this traumatic video. As we looked to our guide for direction, he broke the silence and said that all had been worked out and we would be escorted off the mountain by the military, no doubt with our money paving the escape road ahead. With this announcement, we dug into our food—no knives, forks, or spoons needed—and ate like wild animals. The terror of the past day behind me, I tried to forget what I had seen and heard on that video, but nothing I could do then, or since, can wipe away that memory. Our journey off the mountain later that evening was in silence because we had come to climb a mountain and accomplished our feat, but left with a harsher outlook on humanity as a whole.

Table 6-1   Potential Checklist

Review the following list to see how you can realize your potential.

Realizing Your Potential	Yes	No
Potential		
• Believe that people live life below their potential		
• Measure potential according to a person's IQ		
• Measure potential according to a person's financial status		
• Realize that every action has the potential to change our lives		
• Am able to see the steps needed to realize potential		
• Am able to break routines, make a change, and do something different		
• Am able to move outside my comfort zone and challenge myself		
• Am able to choose a different pathway with unique twists and turns		
• Am able to harness my fear of failure and rejection to take control of life		
• Surround myself with supportive, positive people		

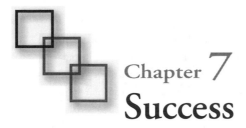

Chapter *7*

Success

Parachutes: Who Packed Yours?

Charles Plumb was a U.S. Navy jet pilot in Vietnam. After 75 combat missions, his plane was destroyed by a surface-to-air missile. Plumb ejected and parachuted into enemy hands. He was captured and spent 6 years in a communist Vietnamese prison. He survived the ordeal and now lectures on lessons learned from that experience. The following is an excerpt from Chapter 16 of his book *Insights into Excellence*.

Recently, I was sitting in a restaurant in Kansas City. A man about two tables away kept looking at me. I didn't recognize him. A few minutes into our meal he stood up and walked over to my table, looked down at me, pointed his finger in my face and said, "You're Captain Plumb."

I looked up and I said, "Yes sir, I'm Captain Plumb."

He said, "You flew jet fighters in Vietnam. You were on the aircraft carrier *Kitty Hawk*. You were shot down. You parachuted into enemy hands and spent six years as a prisoner of war."

I said, "How in the world did you know all that?"

He replied, "Because, I packed your parachute."

I was speechless. I staggered to my feet and held out a very grateful hand of thanks. This guy came up with just the proper words. He grabbed my hand, he pumped my arm and said, "I guess it worked."

"Yes sir, indeed it did," I said, "and I must tell you I've said a lot of prayers of thanks for your nimble fingers, but I never thought I'd have the opportunity to express my gratitude in person."

He said, "Were all the panels there?"

"Well sir, I must shoot straight with you," I said, "of the eighteen panels that were supposed to be in that parachute, I had fifteen good ones. Three were torn, but it wasn't your fault, it was mine. I jumped out of that jet fighter at a high rate of speed, close to the ground. That's what tore the panels in the chute. It wasn't the way you packed it."

"Let me ask you a question," I said, "do you keep track of all the parachutes you pack?"

"No" he responded, "it's enough gratification for me just to know that I've served."

I didn't get much sleep that night. I kept thinking about that man. I kept wondering what he might have looked like in a Navy uniform—a Dixie cup hat, a bib in the back and bell bottom trousers. I wondered how many times I might have passed him on board the *Kitty Hawk*. I wondered how many times I might have seen him and not even said "good morning," "how are you," or anything because, you see, I was a fighter pilot and he was just a sailor. How many hours did he spend on that long wooden table in the bowels of that ship weaving the shrouds and folding the silks of those chutes? I could have cared less… until one day my parachute came along and he packed it for me.

So the philosophical question here is this: How's your parachute packing coming along? Who looks to you for strength in times of need? And perhaps, more importantly, who are the special people in your life who provide you the encouragement you need when the chips are down? Perhaps it's time right now to give those people a call and thank them for packing your chute.

What is success, and why does everyone want us to succeed in everything that we do? Why do we need to succeed? Why can't we just maintain a certain base level of work, play, and existence instead of trying to succeed? Should we be embarrassed if we don't succeed, and does everyone have the ability to succeed? And just how is success measured? Are my interpretations and expectations related to success different or the same as everyone else's? And if different, why should I live up to someone else's expectations of success when I have my own? According to Merriam-Webster's Collegiate Dictionary, 11th edition, *success* is a "degree or measure of succeeding; a favorable or desirable outcome; the attainment of wealth, favor, or eminence." With these descriptions in mind, it appears that to attain success, it will take some degree of work, and/or extremely good luck.

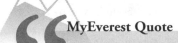

My Travels Through Life

My family's limited financial status while I was growing up challenged my future success. In addition to maintaining our small farm, Dad drove a city bus and each day commuted 60 miles round-trip. Mom stayed at home and held down the fort while Dad worked the land and/or drove the city bus. As the eldest of eight boys and one girl, I can recall that our growing needs exceeded the available resources; even clothes, a basic need, became an expensive commodity. Our pride as children was tempered by the fact that we had to receive community assistance to survive. The lone taxi driver in my hometown of Almonte would drop off used clothes for us on a monthly basis. Each visit was like Christmas, because he would bring a variety of clothes as well as comic books to read. I can fondly remember reading about Archie and Veronica, Casper the Friendly Ghost, and of course my favorites, Superman and Spiderman. We always looked forward to those drop-offs. However, I can recall more than a few occasions when a classmate would ridicule me for wearing a particular type of clothing that their family had donated to the local Catholic Church for the needy. It was embarrassing, but we had little money to purchase new clothes.

I know that my family did everything that they could to make certain that we had what was needed to survive. We had no surplus of toys when we were young, and on those rare occasions when we did receive presents or gifts we very much appreciated them and never threw them away. I believe that being brought up in this environment has helped me to appreciate the needs of those less fortunate. I have learned that you don't have to be wealthy to be happy and that a little of something, anything, if used properly, can go along way. We replaced our clothes when they were threadbare, but we always had mixed emotions about it because we had come to treasure these items.

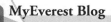

MyEverest Blog

Your mountain is waiting. Go get it. Climb safe, stay strong, be wise. Cheers…—Tony

Fear Is Part of the Puzzle

Challenging my future success as a mountain climber and adventurer was my extreme fear of heights. This first became evident when, as a young child growing up on a farm, I tried to walk on top of the wooden support beams that crisscrossed the upper levels of our huge barn. My brothers and I would spend hours upon hours playing in this barn, exploring the many caverns created by the loose hay, and always ending our play by taking to the support beams at the top of the barn. As winter progressed to spring, the volume of hay was depleted in the barn, which increased the height of these beams from the floor of the barn. Nonetheless, my brothers would run across the beams at full speed and were as agile as the Olympic athletes who compete on the balance beam. But although they transited these beams with little to no fear of the great depths below, I would make my way across by sitting on my butt, legs and arms wrapped around the beam, and pulling myself across very, very slowly. As I moved across these beams, my fear of heights would at times paralyze me to the point where I would have to remain motionless for long periods of time. I can recall during those episodes of paralyzing fear that my heart would race, I would be nauseous, and my thoughts were consumed by my inability to move in any direction for fear of losing my grip. On one occasion, I was actually stranded high on a beam, unknown to my family, and failed to show up for supper. Thanks to a brother's help I was able to get off that beam, and I learned a valuable lesson: make certain that a support system is always available when attempting something very dangerous. However, 50 years later on **Mt. Everest**, I failed to recall that lesson when I found myself in a much more precarious position, with no support system to be found.

Fear is a powerful tool, and I have used it to succeed many times. During a year-long backpacking trip through Latin America in 1993, I had the opportunity to go tandem hang gliding. It was October, and we had been traveling for 10 months and were now in Rio de Janeiro, Brazil. While lying on Pepino Beach, we could not help but see the enormous number of multicolored hang gliders circling high overhead. It was exciting to watch, and we were envious of those flying. As we admired the scene from a distance, we were approached by a local person, who befriended us by offering to drive us to the mountaintop to get a better look at the hang gliders. I was hesitant to go due to my extreme fear of heights, but Carol was anxious to see the city from this vista so we agreed to take the drive to the top of the hill. Once on top, the view was spectacular; we were about 1,700 feet over the city. Below us the tall skyscraper apartment buildings along the beach looked like kids' toys in a sandbox. A wooden ramp led across the parking lot to the edge of the hill, and it was here that the hang gliders got their lift from the winds blowing up the sides of the mountain. With a lot of pressure, reassurance, pushing, prodding, cajoling, and wheeling and dealing, I was eventually persuaded to put on a helmet and get strapped into the rig of the hang glider. The pilot spoke English and explained the routine, which involved three practice runs across the ramp before the actual flight on the fourth run. I told him of my fear of heights, and he seemed sensitive to my fear, but also seemed to ignore it. We ran down the ramp for the first time and stopped at the edge to peer over. The view was nauseating. In the meantime Carol had strapped herself into another rig and was doing practice runs on a parallel ramp in preparation for her test flight. I was still unsure of the whole process and had already ascertained that I could get a ride down the hill to meet Carol on the beach where she would land.

It was time for my second practice, so we started to run down the ramp again, but this time the pilot started to run faster as we approached the halfway point, which was marked with a yellow paint stripe. The red paint stripe, which marked the final edge of the ramp, was approaching rapidly, and my heart started to beat so fast that I could hear it in my ears. What was happening? Why was he running so fast on this second attempt? There was no way we could stop now, or could we? Just 10 feet short of the ramp's edge I stopped running and then did another thing that I was not supposed to do: I grabbed on to the aluminum frame above me. As the edge approached all I can remember is seeing the great expanse below me, my feet suspended in midair, and the speed of our hang glider as we went into a nose dive. All of the other hang gliders that we saw go over the edge had been lifted immediately by the winds, but we were diving down the slope. As our angle corrected we caught the wind, and I started to see blue sky ahead of me instead of the earth racing up to greet me.

I could barely hear my pilot as he yelled some words in Portuguese, and then in English, demanding to know why I had stopped running, and why I had grabbed the frame that had caused our dive. I told him that I thought we had two more practice runs before the real thing, at which point he laughed because he admitted that if we had not taken off then, I would never have consented to go later. It was obvious that he had dealt with other acrophobics and had been successful. We flew for another half hour, and I even took the controls to maneuver us across the sky, crisscrossing in front of Carol and other hang gliders. What a view, what a rush, what an adventure! As we prepared to land, we raced across the beach at what seemed like breakneck speed just a few feet off the surface. Suddenly my pilot flared the nose of the hang glider as he brought the pointed tip of the glider upward, which stalled us and brought us to a stop standing on the beach. Wow, that had been amazing! I looked up at our starting point high up in the sky and was glad that I had not given in to my fear, but had used it to challenge myself to take a risk that I might never had done.

My Journey in Nursing

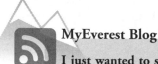

MyEverest Blog

I just wanted to send you my best wishes for nurse's week. Really enjoyed Bo's blog about how we are defined by our experiences and actions of our lifetime. I was thinking about the experiences of the teams of climbers and how you must plan, be prepared, always expect the unexpected, be flexible, and how much smoother things go when you help and support each other. Actually sounds a lot like a shift at work on a patient care unit, or the OR or ER or anywhere else in the hospital.—SD

To be successful, we must be visionary yet focused and passionate yet practical regarding those concerns affecting our professions. My successes as a nurse are the result of hard work, determination, a passion to help others, and a willingness to be both a leader and a team player. I mention a willingness to be a leader because sometimes stepping up to a leadership position can be uncomfortable when you don't feel that you have the capacity to do the job. I can recall my hesitation to become a leader when working as a staff nurse in the operating room at Palmetto Health Richland, despite the support of my nursing leadership. I had been employed in the operating room as a staff nurse for 1 year when the director of surgical services and the manager of the operating room called me to a meeting to discuss the possibility of stepping up to a managerial position. Prior to this position, I already had 10 years of nursing experience in an emergency room where I had functioned as a charge nurse on the evening shift, but there I was competent and comfortable with my surroundings. Here in the operating room, I was struggling to learn the role of the circulator, challenged to learn the names of supplies and equipment for all of the surgical procedures, and still trying to grow as a nurse. While I should have taken the idea of growing into a managerial position as a complement to my potential, instead I took it as a threat because to consider this role meant that I would be competing with veteran operating room nurses who had much more experience and visibility, a few of whom were my mentors as I went through orientation. I queried my director and manager as to why they felt I should be considered for this opportunity.

You Don't Need a Title to Be a Leader

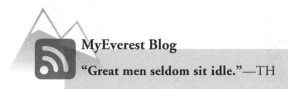

MyEverest Blog

"Great men seldom sit idle."—TH

My director stated that he was not caught up in people needing titles to do what they had to do, and it was for that exact reason that he was considering me for this position. My face must have looked quite puzzled, because he laughed after that statement, which made me feel even more uncomfortable. He then reminded me of my visit to his office six months earlier that he said left a lasting impression. As he recalled, I had been nearing the end of my orientation period and had become quite concerned that there were not enough policies and procedures drafted that correctly identified how we were supposed to perform our jobs as well as use the highly advanced equipment. It was this concern that drove me to his office, but it was my proposed solution that both shocked and impressed him most. My request was to write all new policies and procedures for the entire operating room. To me it didn't appear to be too problematic, but to my director it was a gargantuan task.

With little hesitation other than to ask what I would need, I was given the ultimate responsibility of drafting and updating our policies and procedures. Six months later, after acquiring books on how to write policies and procedures, books on recommended practices, and sample policies and procedures, and after meeting and interviewing our veteran staff who had expertise, my project was completed. We now had well over 200 policies and procedures, all referenced to the recommended practices of our national organization, all in compliance with the demands and expectations of the regulatory agencies, and all ready for dissemination to both old and new staff. For me it had been a "labor of love" because I felt this needed to be done for the safety of the nurses and the patients, and I had not sought any attention or remuneration.

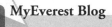

MyEverest Blog

Happy Nurses Week Pat! OK Pat, I had to dig up a Florence quote for you in honor of Nurses Week! This is sooooo true! "The most important practical lesson that can be given to nurses is to teach them what to observe." Florence Nightingale.—SD

No Good Deed Goes Undone

My director had deemed it a very unselfish act and wanted to promote me to a position of leadership. However, because he had developed a system of shared leadership, he was unable to make the final decision alone; I would need to be interviewed by the leadership team just like all of the other applicants. My manager also had prompted me to apply for the role because she, too, had seen my hard work and wanted me to be rewarded with a management position. But although I was flattered that the higher-ups recognized my dedication and hard work, I had to wonder whether I even wanted a managerial position. From my experience, management's every action, every word, and every suggestion are frequently scrutinized, twisted, challenged, and often rejected!

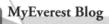

MyEverest Blog

On behalf of the over 5,000 members of the American Organization of Nurse Executives (www.aone.org), we are watching your ascent with many positive thoughts and good wishes. Your efforts in the name of nursing are to certainly be commended! Keep up the great work!—Anonymous

I had worked as a charge nurse in the emergency room and had experienced more than my share of challenges to authority—as well as way too many hassles that were not worth the pay. I explained to both the director and the manager that I was very happy to work behind the scenes and do as much as I could to improve our environment. Their response implied that a lot of improvements could be made by the employee who assumed this position and if I were to be selected, they would support my proposals for change. I did apply for the position, was interviewed, and found out a month later that the job was mine.

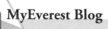

MyEverest Blog

"Anyone can just stand in the spotlight; success goes to the one who makes the spotlight move."—MC

Lateral Violence Occurs at All Levels, to All Sexes, and in All Ways

Through my new position, I found that the leadership role requires focusing and motivating groups to empower and enable them to achieve their goals, as well as knowing how to listen, and being approachable. Unfortunately, my opportunity to develop this fostering relationship was challenged from the onset. Veteran nurses who had applied for the same position had not been given the opportunity to assume this role, and I was now the center of their disdain. A core of veterans created the biggest blockade to my new role by withholding needed information, writing inaccurate reports, and exhibiting a stone-cold attitude. Undaunted, I bit my tongue and set about the task of trying to run a 24-bed surgical suite. My success came slowly. I eventually won over the antagonists through my calm demeanor, fairness, sensitivity to the needs of others, and my way of praising and recognizing staff for jobs well done. I discovered that as a leader you first must know yourself and your environment and, most importantly, be flexible because, similar to climbing a mountain, there are many up and downs, as well as obstacles that get in the way of the summit.

MyEverest Blog

I wanted to let Bonnie's friend know how much I LOVE being a nurse!! I received a BS in Biology and then decided I wanted to go into nursing. I received my BSN from USC in 2002. I couldn't have chosen a better career. The great thing about nursing is there are so many different opportunities. How much direct patient care you want to provide will be determined by where you choose to work.

I was in PACU and ICU where I had continuous direct patient contact. Not only did I get a chance to take care of my patients, but their families as well when they would visit their loved ones. I had the autonomy to provide my patients with the care they needed and took great pride in watching their conditions improve with the decisions I made.

I recently decided I wanted to continue my education and obtain an advanced nursing degree, so I applied to the Nurse Anesthesia program at USC. I have just finished my first semester and love it!! (and still providing hands on care every day I am in clinical!!) Nursing is a wonderful profession… paperwork and all!! You really have the ability to make a difference in your patient's and community's life. Pat is an awesome example of this possibility!!!! The type of care you provide and amount of contact you have with your patient and their family is up to you. Bonnie, I wish your friend the best of luck in whatever career she chooses… I hope it is nursing!!!!!—KG

Time-Out for Surgical Patient Safety

I measure my success in nursing by my ability to make a difference in people's lives. As an elected member of the national board of directors for the Association of periOperative Registered Nurses (AORN), I had the privilege of serving under its president, Bill Duffy. It was Bill's vision that we create a safer perioperative environment for both patients and nurses, and to do so he gathered a board of directors who shared that vision. Together we were able to organize and orchestrate a process that created ripple effects and then quickly gathered momentum to form a wave of patient safety across the United States. This process, called the "Time Out" campaign, highlighted the role of the perioperative nurse in correct site surgery. The time-out process involves the perioperative nurse as a coordinator of a final check before the start of the surgical procedure and verifies with the entire surgical team that they have the correct patient, the correct surgery, and the correct surgical site.

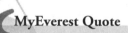

MyEverest Quote

"65% of Sentinel Events are due to a breakdown in basic communication."—The Joint Commission, 2006

This national campaign advised the public of patient safety efforts that were focused on improving the quality of patient care. Thinking outside the box about how to deliver the message of patient safety, we suggested that perioperative nurses develop a collaborative relationship with the risk managers in their hospitals. As a practicing risk manager, I knew that we dealt with incident reports related to safety problems and were responsible for driving the safety efforts within the hospital settings. Risk managers are very aware of the financial losses that hospitals experience on a daily basis related to patient and staff injuries, and they suggest and/or recommend solutions to these problems. However, very few risk managers have ever set foot inside an operating room. The collaborative effort of the Time Out campaign, which brought together AORN, The Joint Commission, ASHRM, ACS, and the Association of Anesthesiologists, demonstrated strength in numbers. It also created a wealth of opportunities for each of the participating organizations. I can remember calling home to Canada on the beginning day of this national campaign to tell my Mom how proud I was to be a part of a campaign that would save the lives of people I would never know.

MyEverest Blog

Sorry I have to catch up on your blogs between working. For some reason there is no stopping babies from being born… even when they are early! :) As far as the facets of nursing,… paperwork will become a thing of the past as computer charting becomes the present as I have been attending more classes to implement more computer based care. Also, my keen interest in nursing informatics keeps me abreast of changes in computerized healthcare.

As a NICU nurse, there is SO much more to what I do than paperwork. Examples of amazing things that I've been a part of are: caring for a baby weighing less than one pound, providing end of life support for infant and his family, hummed and rocked an irritable baby to sleep, advocated for better therapeutic measures for my patients, stood by my position even when the doctor and other nurses didn't see when something was wrong with a patient (That experience validated the "gut" instinct that they teach in nursing school.… I just KNEW something was wrong! PS the baby turned out ok), and the moment that a mother gets to kangaroo her infant for the first time. This is just a few of the experiences that make nursing in a neonatal unit worthwhile!—Anonymous

Summit of Patient Safety

Nursing success as a whole reflects our efforts to effectively reduce patient injuries in a very fast paced, technically demanding healthcare environment. I refer to this effort as reaching the summit of patient safety because it is very similar to reaching a mountaineering summit: it is the culmination of our training, teamwork, proper use of equipment/gear, and leadership that helps get us to the top. Many of the patient safety issues have been related to challenges faced by nurses, such as low staffing levels, long work shifts, look-alike drugs, illegible physician handwriting, and lack of training. A 1999 Institute of Medicine (IOM) report indicates that between 44,000 and 98,000 people die in hospitals each year as a result of preventable medical errors and adding to these challenges is a looming national nurse shortage, projected to be between 800,000 and 1.1 million by 2020.

> **MyEverest Blog**
>
> **"Success is measured by all the work you put into your achievements. What you achieve is a bonus."—MC**

To combat these issues and many more, nurses have helped to create a culture change in health care that includes better teams and teamwork, fewer errors, greater efficiency, and the end result of more positive patient outcomes. According to Dr. Lucian Leape, "Incompetent people are, at most, 1% of the problem. The other 99% are good people trying to do a good job who make very simple mistakes and it's the processes that set them up to make these mistakes."* None of us as nurses intend to harm a patient, but we may inadvertently do so as a result of system issues. We are now focusing more on *what* caused the injury, not *who* caused it. Through use of root cause analysis, enhanced communication, accurate reporting, and process redesign, nurses have been able to significantly reduce the harm caused by mistakes. Additionally, solutions to the nursing shortage have to be addressed and include addressing nursing issues such as the nursing faculty shortage, additional clinical space/opportunities, simulation labs, and creative, innovative academic/service partnerships.

It's That "Giving Back" Time in Life

> **MyEverest Blog**
>
> **I am not a nurse yet—only a second-semester nursing student at the age of 36 years. I work as a CNA in a hospital. Nursing is so much more than paperwork. Nursing is so many things. Nursing is assessing patients to determine their current health status, it is communicating with the patients about their needs now and in the future, nursing is about educating, nursing is about making sure the patient is safe and educated once they leave the healthcare facility. Nursing is putting patients on bedpans and making sure they have enough intake of fluids. Nursing is about changing beds and making patients comfy. Nursing is about caring and caring some more. Without nurses, the doctors would be lost, for the nurses are the ones that are constantly caring and monitoring the patients at the bedside. Nursing is much more than this. Nurses are so needed and I am so happy that someday I will be able to say to the next person, "I am a nurse."—GG**

---

*Leape, L. L. (2001). *How many medical deaths are there really?* Retrieved March 18, 2009, from http://www.aspf.org/resource_center/newsletter/2001/fall/03errors.htm

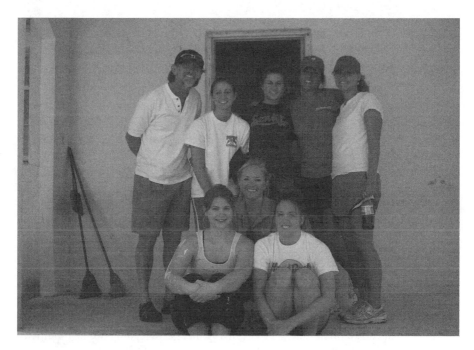

Success for me has been the opportunity to give back to society. Many people feel this same compulsion: they consider it a way to live a meaningful life through their attempts to make a difference in others' lives. True satisfaction and meaning in life are derived from making a positive change in an area about which you are most passionate, and in my case I am passionate about nursing, but more specifically the opportunity to teach nursing students about the joys of nursing! Nurses are always giving of themselves. They volunteer for committees, are involved in their communities, and give their time and money to help those in need. All of us contribute in some way or another because our goals are to change things for the better. My passion for teaching extends outside the classroom: I typically extend myself quite often to help students in need of direction, jobs, guidance, and support.

MyEverest Blog

Thanks for giving the detailed directions on how to donate for your cause! I feel much better now that I have actually donated something to this. I'm not sure how long they will keep that open but as I can afford, I will contribute to it! I think if you can make the sacrifices you're making, certainly we can. Most of us in our lifetime will benefit from the services of a nurse and I personally would like to make sure more are trained!—BI

MyEverest Blog

Hey Pat. I just wanted you to know that my husband and I contributed to your worthy cause. Many in my family were and are both doctors and nurses (except for me ... I'm too squeamish) so we realize how important your cause is to many who desire to become nurses.—RM

My Climbs on the Mountains

Success in mountain climbing can mean many things to many people, but for most it seems to be a successful summit. To say that mountain climbers are competitive is a great understatement; they do not strive to compete against others but against themselves as they push the limits of extreme adventure and physical conditioning. However, the finish line for climbers is not the summit—that is only half the competition. The true completion of the successful challenge comes at the base of the climb, because coming down often provides more of a challenge than going up the mountain. On **Mt. Everest**, it has been estimated that approximately 80% of those that die do so on the descent, because this is when the biggest challenge to physical and mental conditioning exists.

7 Summits of the World: A Team Effort

I attribute my success climbing the 7 Summits of the World to many factors, but the most important was the team factor. On all of the mountains teams were a crucial part of success, and being a good team member meant a better chance of a positive climb. As an independent climber, on each climb I was introduced to total strangers from all over the world. Even though we had a common interest in making a successful summit, we all had a diversity of experiences, languages, and cultures. Additionally, we were all motivated in different ways: some were much more positive than others, and those who lacked motivation tended to reduce the effectiveness of the team. As teammates we all lived by the acronym TEAM: Together Each Achieves More. In a very short time, we had to learn to be friends and try to understand the strengths and weaknesses of each team member.

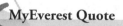

MyEverest Quote

"You cannot be a good mountaineer, however great your ability, unless you are cheerful and have the spirit of good comradeship. Friends are as important as achievement. Another is that teamwork is the one key to success and that selfishness only makes a man small. Still another is that no man, on a mountain or elsewhere, gets more out of anything than he puts into it."—Tenzing Norgay

Teamwork on the mountain is as crucial to success as it is in the hospital system. Motivation to do your work is just as critical in the hospital because job satisfaction and motivation are so highly correlated.

Getting Up Is Only Half the Challenge

My success in the mountains has come from hard work, extensive training, and a strong determination to return home safely. But many factors challenged my desire for success: my fear of heights, extreme weather, and poorly trained climbers. In order to become a mountain climber, as in becoming a nurse, you need to train. You must learn skills to accomplish tasks, and it takes time to learn those skills. Practice through return demonstration (teaching what you have just learned) and hands-on training provide a higher level of self-esteem. You have no doubt heard the adage "Practice makes perfect." Well, it applies to both nursing and mountain climbing. Education experts note that it takes multiple repetitions of a task before it is learned, with this subsequent mastering of skills preparing the nurse, or climber, for more complicated tasks. Just think about how complicated it would be for a nurse to care for a postoperative open-heart patient as his or her very first patient, which would be similar to climbing **Mt. Everest** as your very first mountain. Both would be disasters just waiting to happen. However, success is not always measured by reaching the summit; getting down off the mountain safely is often the true measure of success.

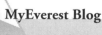

MyEverest Blog

Just remember now you're up there—don't stuff up the landing... cheers—and well done...—clarky

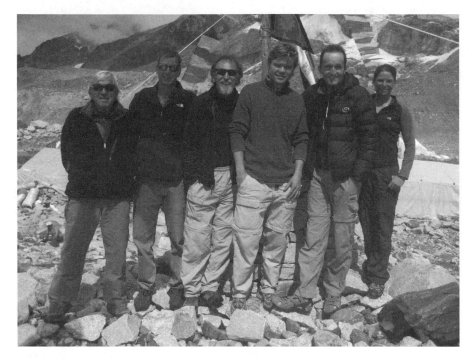

I learned this lesson the hard way on almost all the mountains I have climbed, because each descent proved more challenging than the ascent. The adrenaline rush of making the summit lasts only so long: soon after, the fatigue of sleepless nights, the lack of nutrition and hydration, and the realization that there is a long way to go to reach high camp all set in. My fear of heights was challenged on each mountain, but on three—**Mt. McKinley** in Alaska, **Carstensz Pyramid** in Indonesia, and **Mt. Everest** in Nepal—that fear was almost paralyzing.

MyEverest Blog

"Success may be found when you reach the top of the mountain but lucky is the one who finds adventure along the way."—MC

The Ups and Downs

Mt. McKinley is my favorite of the 7 Summits of the World, because it is a true winter wonderland. Once you land at Base Camp on the Kahiltna Glacier, you leave the greenery, rivers, and flora and fauna behind and are faced with a bright white backdrop of ice, glacier, and snow. The final ridge climb to the summit was what concerned me most on this mountain. To deal with the vertical drops on each side of the narrow ledge, I adopted a shuffling movement, slowly sliding my feet along the surface of the snow. I actually had to be comforted by my guide before I transited this final pitch, because my fear of heights had gotten the best of me and I had been reduced to tears. Compounding this summit attempt was the fact that the wind was blowing very strongly and the rope that connected me to the climber in front was actually lifted off the ground and kept taut in midair. Because of this wind, I had to overcorrect my body alignment to lean into the wind, which pushed me closer to the edge. Despite my fear of heights, I was able to accomplish a successful summit bid because of a team effort: on this mountain, we were roped to one another and collectively were able to summit as a team.

MyEverest Blog

Go hard, don't look down until you are on the top.—MC

Carstensz Pyramid, my fifth of the 7 Summits, brought my fear of heights to a new level: rock climbing the 3,000-foot rock face approach demanded climbing skills that were far superior to what I possessed. This meant total open exposure, and the fear was simply paralyzing. Due to political unrest, no one had legally climbed this mountain in three years, and we were the first team to reopen it to the climbing world. Our summit push took place at night, so the exposure of the rock face did not bother me as much as it would the next dawn. But even in the dark, I could still feel and imagine the wide open expanse far below me. Rock face successfully scaled, I still had major challenges to my fear of heights because I had to traverse gaping chasms and more vertical walls. I reverted to creeping along some of the perilous ledges on my hands and feet and had to endure scorn and ridicule from my fellow climbers, because they did not think I could make it to the top if I had to crawl. I proved them wrong because I did summit. Summit reached, I celebrated, but that was short-lived because I now had to rappel down the 3,000 feet of exposed vertical rock face in the daylight.

MyEverest Quote

"My success evolved from working hard at the business at hand every day."—Johnny Carson

Freezing cold, exhaustion, dehydration, and malnourishment were conditions that challenged me as I started my descent. As I rappelled down the face of this cliff, I took time to make certain that the safety lines, harness, and carabiners were secured and in proper functioning order. In the beginning, I kept my gaze on the rock face directly in front of me, not looking left, right, or down, but halfway through the descent I worked up the courage to stop in midair and take in the majesty of the scenery all around me. I'll never forget the moment: I slowly looked to my left and then my right and finally directly below me. Suspended at 1,500 feet, secured to a rock face, the breathtaking view all around me was priceless. I was secure in my faith that the harness and ropes would prevent me from falling. That faith was soon tested, because moments later I actually rappelled off the rope on my second-to-last pitch of the descent. Our climb pushed us and the ropes to the limit, and unfortunately in this case the rope could not take the strain. The ropes had been weakened by years of weather, and a knot at the rope's end had frayed away. My fall seemed like slow motion as I helplessly watched the rope's end floating away above me. Before my brain could decipher what had happened, my body slammed onto a rock ledge 20 feet below. My helmet absorbed the head trauma while my backpack cushioned the body blow.

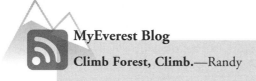

MyEverest Blog

Climb Forest, Climb.—Randy

I remember lying there, staring up at the rock face and marveling that I had just successfully descended that large granite rock. Or had I? Initially stunned, with the wind knocked out of me, I fought to catch my breath. This brush with death I will never, ever forget. Slowly I attempted to wiggle my fingers and toes to see if the pounding pain in my back indicated a spinal fracture. Fingers moved, as did toes. What a relief! I lay there for what seemed like hours and just looked up at the clouds scurrying across the sky, glad to be alive. Reflecting on what had just happened, I cursed myself. I should have taken more care and inspected the weathered ropes more closely. I slowly rose to my feet, and the pain in my back felt like I had been stabbed. But, hey, I was alive and walking, albeit with a limp. My faith in my climbing skills had been challenged, but I had persevered and now had successfully surmounted my fears and this daunting rock face. I was able to accomplish this, despite imperfections with the system, which is not unlike the challenges that we face in our hospital systems.

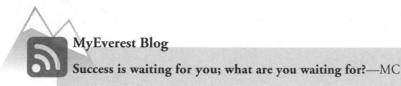

MyEverest Blog

Success is waiting for you; what are you waiting for?—MC

Enjoying the Journey

Mt. Everest challenged my fear of heights like nothing else has on this earth, and I suppose that is only fitting because **Mt. Everest** is the highest mountain in the world. The Khumbu Icefall, with its ladder crossings over bottomless crevasses, and Summit Day, from Camp 4 to the top of the world, were each very perilous. The Khumbu Icefall, a 2,000-foot-tall shifting river of ice made up of crevasses, ladders, steep inclines, and constant twists and turns, is an infamous labyrinth! My biggest fear on the lower part of the mountain was crossing crevasses on multiple aluminum ladders that were strapped together and secured into the ice.

From Base Camp to Camp 1 at the top of the Khumbu Icefall, there are at least 40 ladder crossings, each as demanding as the next. We were extremely attentive to safety precautions on each crossing, because a slip or fall could be life ending. At one point, I did fall off a vertical ladder that was not well secured and was very fortunate that a snow bridge in the middle of the crevasse arrested my fall. Had it not been there, I would have been okay—just suspended by a safety line over a 200-foot crevasse! Higher up the mountain my fear of heights was challenged on Summit Day by the extreme vertical drops: 10,000 feet into Nepal on one side and 12,000 feet into Tibet on the other side. Adherence to strict protocol on use of carabiners to clip in/out of safety lines, awareness of location, pacing of rhythm, and trust in the safety line system made for a safe journey, despite the fact that I would not look down!

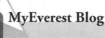

MyEverest Blog

Pat, you amaze me! You are a climbing machine! Never mind ALL the obstacles that you faced—wind, cold, oxygen mask, being a little over age 30, etc., etc.—nothing seemed to faze you—just "we went to this camp or that"—"we're headed for the summit"—almost just like (yawn) another day at the office! No wonder you just completed the 7 summits! All I can say is "I tip my hat" to you, sir! And, if I ever need a good nurse I'll bet I know who to call!!! —J

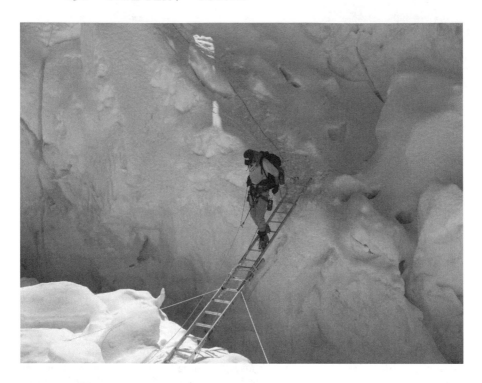

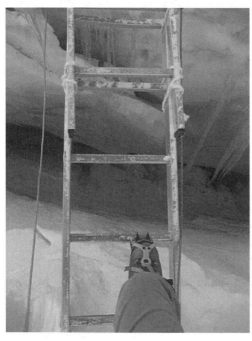

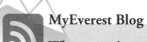

MyEverest Blog

What a testimony to personal dedication, strength, encouragement, love and commitment you have shown us. Thanks for sharing this blog with us so that we can all experience your special moment.—Paula

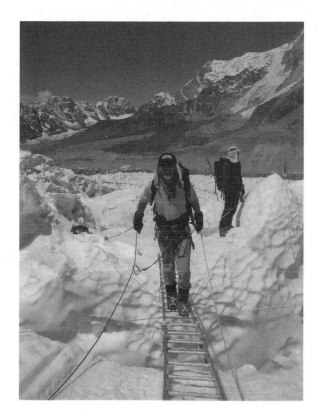

Table 7-1 Success Checklist

Review the following list to see how you can succeed.

Realizing Your Success	Yes	No
Success		
• Able to picture your future If you can see it, you can get there		
• Accept that success is a matter of small, single steps on a daily basis		
• Realize that it's the little choices you make each day that can lead to success		
• Accept that every opportunity leads to a door opening		
• Realize that each trail is an opportunity for change, success		
• Realize that fear of what is down the trail can be a motivator to success		
• Accept that success does not require superhuman strength or super intelligence		
• Have confidence to succeed		
• Surround self with positive people		

Realizing Your Success	Yes	No
Success		
• Make contacts with inspirational people		
• Are willing to take a risk and get outside your comfort zone		
• Are willing to change habits to succeed		
• Have motivators pushing you to succeed		
• Realize that if you keep doing everything that you have always done in the past, you will keep getting the same results		
• Realize that once you take the first step, you will never be the same		
• Scare yourself by thinking of the financial cost of attaining success		
• Realize that the right attitude can make the difference between success and failure		
• Use the fear of regret to succeed		
• Feel that you control your environment and live life by choice and not chance		

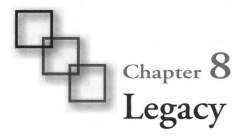

Chapter 8
Legacy

A few years ago, at the Seattle Special Olympics, nine contestants, all physically or mentally disabled, assembled at the starting line for the 100-yard dash. At the gun, they all started out, not exactly in a dash, but with a relish to run the race to the finish and win. All, that is, except one little boy who stumbled on the asphalt, tumbled over a couple of times, and began to cry. The other eight heard the boy cry. They slowed down and looked back, then they all turned around and went back—every one of them. One girl with Down syndrome bent down and kissed him and said, "This will make it better." Then all nine linked arms and walked together to the finish line. Everyone in the stadium stood. The cheering went on for several minutes. People who were there are still telling the story. Why? Because deep down we know this one thing: what matters in this life is more than winning for ourselves. What matters in this life is helping others win, even if it means slowing down and changing our course.

—Anonymous

What is legacy, and how do we get it? Do all of us have the potential to leave a legacy, and if so does it have to be monetary? According to *Merriam-Webster's Collegiate Dictionary*, 11th edition, *legacy* is "a gift of monies or property," or "something transmitted by or received from an ancestor or predecessor or from the past." The meaning that I intend to build on is that of something immaterial, as a style of philosophy that is passed from one generation to another. In other words, legacy is that personal impact that influences the future of those around us. It is sometimes very easy to see the impact from those who are in highly visible positions, such as presidents, actors, and spiritual leaders, but we, too, have the capacity to leave our own legacy. Just take a moment to think of the many family members who have impacted our lives, the various teachers who have encouraged and inspired us, and our friends and neighbors who influenced us to be better people. Our own personal legacy can be something tangible, such as money, property, or even an artistic creation like a video that will express our views and sentiments for future generations, or it may be intangible, such as the time and effort we donated to a charity or cause that has been a priority in our lives.

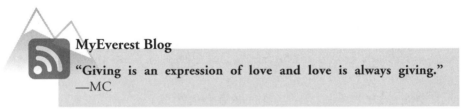

MyEverest Blog

"Giving is an expression of love and love is always giving."
—MC

My Travels Through Life

When I look back on life, and I do that quite often now, I am always amazed at where I am and how I got to be here. Was it a comedy of errors, six degrees of separation, inevitable or fate? Did I travel a path less trodden for a reason, and how did I find my way? Were there markers along the way as on a trail through the woods, or was there deep brush ahead with no clear view of what was to happen or where to go? I have always heard and maintained that things in life happen for a reason. But is this really true? Once something has happened, it seems like we can always go back and find a trail that leads to that eventual outcome, or is that just a way of rationalizing that what happens in life does so for a reason? And, if that were the case, we should be able to forecast everything that will happen in our lives. However, to quote Robert Burns, "The best laid schemes of mice and men gang aft agley" (often paraphrased "'The best-laid plans of mice and men go oft awry"): no matter what we plan and put in place, there will always be uncertainty and surprise. Yet, along the way there are signs or markers that should give a hint of the future and what is in store. Have we not commented on a gifted child who is able to play a musical instrument so superbly at an early age and known for certain that this gift would give him direction in life by opening doors to opportunity?

Growing to Our Maximum Potential

This situation described is most obvious and the signs very clear, but what do we make of those signs that are less clear but just as helpful? And who is able to take note of those signs and realize the potential? Surely it is crucial that parents note the telltale signs of growth, development, and socialization, but what should we make of the signs that are less telling, such as the dreams of a child who imagines adventure, exploration, and risk taking as his future? And who should notice these dreams as they are played out in the schoolyards, tree forts, and back alleys of a community, away from a parent's sight and therefore unsupported by family?

As I look back at life now, those signs of what I would become loom larger than billboard ads, yet at the time they were but a chance happening, a dream, and not even something I myself noticed. Today, it is simply a matter of connecting the trail markers to see the path that led to where I now stand. The path, as I see it, was wrought with challenge, despair, and adversity; yet along the way there were forks in the trail that led to hope, enlightenment, and reward.

To manage this path of life, I had to rely on the legacy left by family and friends, as a hiker would rely on a map. They gave me guidance and direction when I could not find the way. My sustenance along the path was my deeply rooted religious beliefs and faith in a higher being. It was this faith that kept me going when things got tough, and things did get tough! My shelter and protection from the elements was my inner calm that held me fast as storms raged around me. This inner calm arose after years of self-doubt and has been a salvation. And finally, it was the love of a woman, who became a wife and best friend, and who joined me on the trail of life to give me companionship and love. Without this final piece, I would be lost in the woods, with little to no direction. Looking back, the path is clear, yet that isn't it always the case.

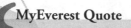

MyEverest Quote

"I believe that every human has a finite number of heartbeats. I don't intend to waste any of mine."—Neil Armstrong

I was born in Ottawa, Ontario, on a blustery winter day. My birth heralded a wintry storm that shut down the city. Mom remembers the challenges of getting me home from the hospital; perhaps this was a sign that I was meant to be there? Memories of my earliest years are composed of just a few tattered black-and-white photos coupled with supporting tales from Mom and Dad. The photos always show a smiling toddler accompanied by a man in uniform who is very thin, very tall, and also smiling. I was the first of what would become Bernard and Rita's litter of nine children. No wonder he was smiling. I, his firstborn, had his middle name, Patrick. What a great way to start a family, or so it seemed. When I look at those photos, I see an old family car, my mom, and even Grandma is there because when I was born we lived in her home. Mom and Dad had married late in life, and to save money they lived with her mother. Mom worked in the government as an administrative clerk and made a minimal wage. Dad was a bus driver and worked long and hard because he took his profession very seriously. At retirement, he'd accumulated 35 years of accident-free driving, a feat unheard of today! Both were very frugal, and these were lessons well learned.

Mom and Dad were happy with the city and had lots of friends, but they were given an opportunity to move to the country and live on a farm owned by my grandpa, Dad's father. This small country town, Almonte, was 30 miles away from the city, and Dad had been devoting all his spare time to helping Grandpa with the farm because he was getting older and was not able to manage on his own. The work on the farm challenged my dad as he committed long hours to both jobs and had a lot of driving to do in between. My brothers and I inherited this same work ethic as we all seem to be driven to do more than is required, always without complaint.

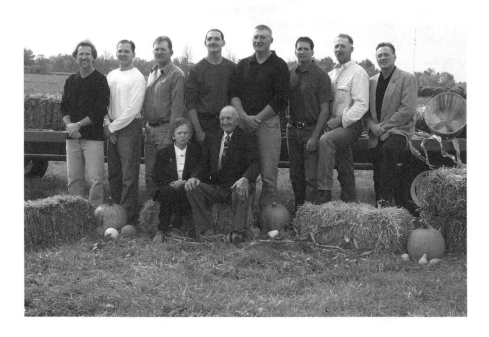

While Dad wrestled with managing two jobs, a recent move from the city to a country farm, and the challenges of family life, I unknowingly began to learn from his trials and tribulations. Growing up in a small farming community was very simple, yet fundamental, and I now see that my present-day values were honed in that setting. I learned the lessons of the farm, the value of a community, the strength of religion, and the dedication of friends. All of these were very inspirational and instilled within me a desire to help others.

Inspiring others is not something that we normally set out to do consciously, but it happens sometimes when we least expect it. While backpacking around the world for a year in 1988 and in Latin America for a year in 1993, I wrote a column for my hometown newspaper. The column, "Letters Home," was a travelogue of our adventures. I listed each country we visited and included historical, geographical, and tourist-related details, along with pictures and maps. It was a labor of love because I wanted to share my experiences with as many people as possible. For some, reading the articles would be a déjà vu experience, whereas for others it would be something new that they had never heard of, or maybe they had heard of it and wanted to learn more. On return from our round-the-world trip, we met with a couple in my hometown who had not only read the articles, but had highlighted segments, made notes, and had done some further research into the areas noted. Jim and June's dream had been to do what we had done, but they did not know how to do it. They were a few years older than Carol and I and had not backpacked, or stayed in youth hostels, or hitchhiked, but they wanted to learn. After days of visiting with them and sharing our maps, diaries, places to go and things to see, we parted company. Six months later, Jim and June took off on the same trip as we had and started to send us postcards from places we had visited all over the world. We were able to live their trip vicariously through them, as they had done through us earlier. After our backpacking trip through Latin America, we again shared our details with Jim and June, after which they took off on the same trip. Of course, as they traveled more on each trip, they blossomed out to find new and unique experiences that we never had.

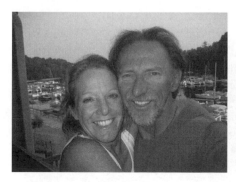
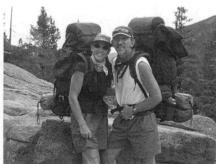

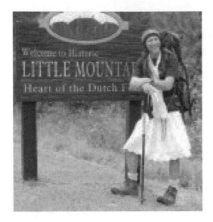

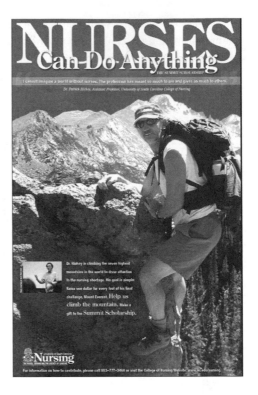

Again, on **Mt. Everest** I was able to inspire and mentor through my 2-month-long blog. The 700 pages of text from that blog show the great number of people who learned about not only the challenges of mountain climbing but, more importantly, the challenges of nursing. The media attention—in the form of magazines, books, newspapers, radio, and journals at the local, state, and national levels—both before and after my climb of **Mt. Everest** has elicited many requests for information, as well as support for the Summit Scholarship. As I tell my students constantly, behind every door is an opportunity that you will never expect. However, you first have to open that door.

MyEverest Blog

The title of this piece is called "Who Am I??"

This is a question that has been on my mind (and perhaps many fellow climbers') numerous times throughout the 2007 Everest Expedition.

Who am I? This question appears at interesting times: while dangling from a rope, crossing a ladder over a bottomless crevasse, dodging avalanches, seeing a dead body being carried down the

mountain, climbing through the Khumbu Icefall in the early morning and hoping a chunk of ice the size of a house doesn't decide
to fall and crush me, climbing the seemingly vertical Lhotse face
where rocks and ice fall violently and erratically right toward me, or
simply lying in my tent—during these exciting, hectic and tranquil
times I ask myself, "Who Am I?"

I have been thinking deeply about this simple yet perplexing
question.

After a proper period of reflection, it became apparent to me that I
was not just a name, not just a brother, not just a son, not just a someday father or husband, not just a climber, not just a businessman.

I discovered that it is a fundamental flaw to define ourselves by
our physical presence. This is because our physical attributes are
consistently regenerating.

The human body pretty much regenerates itself every year; some
organs grow faster than others. Hair continues to grow no matter how often we cut it (for most of us, anyway), and the skin we
sport today was not there six months ago. Nor will it be with you
six months from now. Even your internal organs slowly die and
rebuild.

So if we aren't entirely defined by our physical attributes or the
name we give ourselves, how are we defined? Some believe we are
defined by a spirit or by the spirituality that guides the decisions
we make in life. I think that approach is part of the answer, but I
think there's more.

"We are defined by the experiences and actions of our lifetime."

We are defined by years of fun and boredom, of excitement and
terror, of pleasure and pain, of love and loathing. Some portion of
the weathering and scars is visible. Some of it lies much deeper. We
are defined by the friends we have kept as well as those we elected not
to. We are a product of the things we controlled as well as the stuff
that landed on our laps courtesy of fate, chance, bad luck, or destiny.

Now I ask you (the audience)—who are you?—Bo Parfet

My Journey in Nursing

What is our legacy as nurses? Do we want to be remembered as "Super Nurses," do we
want to change the world, or do we want to be part of the team to cure cancer? Or is
our legacy that nurses can do anything? I firmly believe that each and every one of us,
as nurses, has created a legacy for others to follow, whether we know it or not. Most of

us have had a "calling" to our profession, and all of us want to make a difference in our patients' lives. The best legacy is to lead whenever we can, and I believe that we do have that opportunity to lead every day whether as a nurse manager in a hospital, as a member of a community committee, or as the head of a family. People lead for a variety of reasons, but the common denominator of most leaders is a passion for life and what they do. Leadership requires a wide range of skills, techniques, and strategies, such as the ability to plan and communicate effectively and an awareness of the wider environment in which the team operates. To keep the team together, the leader is responsible for ensuring that goals are established and met, and the team is cohesive and happy.

I believe that the true test of leadership is the ability to lead. How many people would follow us, or take our commands, if we did not have an official title as a leader, or if we could neither reward nor penalize? If this were the case, how many of us could truly say that we are leaders? Part of the solution is in how we do our jobs. When we do our jobs with initiative and determination to make a positive difference, we become leaders.

Touching the Future

MyEverest Blog

I've been following your progress and am in complete awe of what you guys are doing. I've taken the liberty of forwarding your blog address and instructions for donating to the scholarship to my mom and sister, both are nurses. I have asked they forward it to everyone. I also made a donation to your cause. I understand the need for nurses and the impending shortage. The care given to me by some amazing nurses five years ago made it possible for me to win my own battle and still be here today. The doctors helped, too… but the nurses… they are always there for you.—CH

My good friend Bill Duffy was the national president of the Association of periOperative Registered Nurses (AORN) from 2004 to 2006, and during that time created his own legacy as a caring leader with a vision of creating positive outcomes for surgical patients. Bill coordinated a national campaign called "Time Out" and has saved countless lives through his development of a safer perioperative environment. In creating his legacy, Bill said it best in one of his speeches: "The care you provide touches not only the patient … but the patient's family, children, and the future of their children's children.…" If we could create a legacy, what more could we aspire to do than that of making a difference in others' lives? I truly believe that all of us have the potential to make a difference every day—through coaching and mentoring, or by our actions on committees and work with charities, or by listening to a friend, opening a door for a person, or smiling at a stranger.

MyEverest Blog

What a wonderful posting—Who am I? Very thought provoking and insightful. We are defined in many ways by our experiences and the people we meet along the way. We must always remember that the even the little things we share with others can have a big impact on their lives. The question—Who am I?—is one I would like to visit (or revisit) often! Thanks!—Anonymous

When I speak of the future and the lives that we touch, I am always reminded of my favorite movie, *It's a Wonderful Life*. I love the message: George Bailey is shown what a difference he has made in the lives of others. Unfortunately, we don't have the opportunity to have a guardian angel, like Clarence was in the movie, to help us to see what a difference we can, and do, make. A simple reflection of what we have done in our nursing careers, and the volume of lives that we have touched, should reinforce for all of us the legacy of caring that we have left behind. As nurses, just think of how many lives we have touched, how many hands we have held, how many tears we have dried, how much pain we have relieved, how much comfort we have brought to dying patients, and how many lives we have brought into this world. For those who are students and/or those who are just starting as nurses, our future depends on you. Know that you, too, will make a difference in the life of each patient that you touch, with your hands and your heart. Just think of how many lives you will affect, how many babies you will hold, and how you can make such a difference in the lives of others … and you get paid to do this!

MyEverest Blog

Hi Pat, today is International Nurses Day in New Zealand! Probably the rest of the world tomorrow because of the date change. All nurses in Auckland received fresh fruit kebabs just to remind us of the day and the multicultural aspect of nursing.—WA

Saving Lives

When I was in high school and troubled about what to do with my life, a guidance counselor directed me to attend a presentation by a local college on a career as a nurse. Hesitantly I attended this meeting, but while there I learned a lot about nursing. One thing that surprised me most was that nurses can save lives. Up until that point, I had thought that this was exclusively part of a doctor's role. I remember that this was a powerful moment: it was one of the main reasons that I became a nurse ... to save lives. Don Berwick, MD, MPP, President and CEO of the Institute for Healthcare Improvement, summed it up best as follows: "The names of the patients whose lives we can save can never be known. Our contribution will be what did not happen to them. And, though they are unknown, we will know that mothers and fathers are at graduations and weddings that they would have missed, and that grandchildren will know grandparents they might never have known, and holidays will be taken, and work completed, and books read, and symphonies heard, and gardens tended that, without our work, would never have been."

Mr. Berwick has orchestrated the 100,000 Lives Campaign, which strives to make health care safer and more effective with the overarching goal of ensuring that hospitals attain positive outcomes for all patients. This campaign has since escalated to become the 5 Million Lives Campaign. Nurses are an integral part of this campaign. We have been able to initiate many of the campaign steps such as deployment of rapid response teams, prevention of adverse drug effects, and prevention of surgical site infections. Through the introduction of best practices and evidence-based practice, nurses have been able to create better outcomes for patients.

Summit Scholarship Speaking Tour

MyEverest Blog

I challenge my old friends (and dear friends) at Palmetto Health and my peers at USC College of Nursing to take the opportunity to donate to the future of Nursing. As we all know, many of us are nearing the age of "slowing down, or skipping out the door to an easier, less stressful lifestyle." We have to share our knowledge and wisdom to those who will follow us and mentor them as they develop. Let us make their pathways to professional nursing nicer than the ones we have had.—MW

The opportunity to be a spokesperson for nursing, and in doing so to be able to advocate for students and their financial needs, has been a blessing. Audience after audience at my presentations has acknowledged the need for nurses: individuals have recounted their positive experiences with nurses and have praised nursing as the most honorable of professions. Many nurses in attendance, both working and retired, echo the need for more nurses within our profession and lament one of our greatest hurdles in the profession, the shrinking acceptance rates of nursing programs at the college level due to the shortage of nursing faculty.

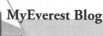

MyEverest Blog

What you are doing for the nursing profession as a whole is absolutely phenomenal. You are definitely practicing what Dr. Mary Wakefield suggests and that is to wear your profession like a badge of honor. What an honor it is for all of us to follow and share your successes!—CAC

The goal of the Summit Scholarship at the University of South Carolina, developed just prior to my departure for **Mt. Everest** in March 2007, was to raise $1.00 for every foot of **Mt. Everest**'s altitude, which is 29,035 feet. In order to be an endowed scholarship for student nurse use, a minimum of $25,000 needs to be accrued. The speaking tour has taken me to gatherings of community and civic groups, physicians, lawyers, and students from grade school to university. I have spoken at corporate meetings and led exercises in teamwork as well as communication. At each and every meeting, I speak of the challenges in nursing and how those in attendance can make a difference.

Most recently, I have initiated a second nursing scholarship called the Nurses Can Do Anything Scholarship. This scholarship will be provided through the National Student Nurses Association (NSNA) and again to be endowed requires a minimum of $25,000. All monies received from the sale of this book as well as all monies from speaking fees and honoraria go directly to these two scholarships. I am hopeful that more scholarships for student nurses can be developed, because there are never enough scholarships to meet the need.

Some of my most memorable presentations have been at the primary and middle school levels, and it truly has been a joy to meet these kids who are sponges for education. Some of these schools regularly followed my blog on **Mt. Everest** and had a real-life opportunity to dialogue with a climber facing the biggest challenge of his life. Four of those schools that I was able to visit were St. Mary's in Almonte, Ontario; Oake

Pointe Elementary in Columbia, South Carolina; Wilson Hall in Sumter, South Carolina; and Saluda Trail Middle School in Rock Hill, South Carolina. At each school, I shared lessons learned on the mountain and taught both students and teachers how to apply them to their daily lives. I was given a list of over 50 questions prior to my visit at Wilson Hall and was quite impressed with the questions students came up with, such as: how long does it take to train for a climb and what kind of training do you do; have you ever felt scared that you might lose your life; what was it like to know that if you completed **Mt. Everest** you would meet your goal; and did you have fun? These were quite interesting questions from a group of very bright students. What excited me most about these school presentations though were the letters and comments that I received from students and teachers.

MyEverest Blog

Here are some notes from primary and middle school students:

Dear Dr. Patrick Hickey, Thank you for inspiring me to believe in myself and overcome my fears.—SW (Oake Pointe Elementary)

Dear Dr. Hickey, You've inspired me a lot to achieve my dreams. You remind me of Indiana Jones because he is a teacher but also does all this cool stuff just like you as a nurse, but you do REALLY COOL STUFF! I just wanted to let you know how much you changed my way of thinking about what I can't do.—MB (Oake Pointe Elementary)

Dear Dr. Hickey, Everybody tells me that I can do everything ... I believe now that I know it is true.—LLA (Wilson Hall)

Dear Dr. Hickey, I really learned a lot when you came, like how a person from anywhere around the world can set their goals in life and succeed with the help and support of their friends and family. —BK (Wilson Hall)

Dear Dr. Hickey, You really did inspire me with goal setting, the attitude of just never giving up, and just having fun at it. Also, like you, I have acrophobia ... and who knows I just might climb the seven summits, or be an acrobat, or fly an airplane.—RR (Wilson Hall)

Dear Dr. Hickey, My mom was amazed when I told her everything you had done and what you taught us. I now believe that anyone can follow their dreams and anyone can conquer their fears. You may not be Superman, but you are a hero to me.—MS (Wilson Hall)

Dear Dr. Hickey, It's so amazing that you overcame your fear of heights and climbed the seven tallest mountains in the world. I couldn't believe that I shook your hand. I really look up to your bravery, confidence, and achievements.—E (Wilson Hall)

Dear Dr. Hickey, You taught me that you need to set (and keep) goals. I always set goals, but never keep them. You also taught me to confront my fears.—L (Wilson Hall)

Dear Dr. Hickey, I enjoyed all the stories you shared with us and you inspired me. If you can climb the seven summits then I can follow my dreams to be president. You are the best!—MH (Wilson Hall)

Dear Dr. Hickey, Although it seems difficult, you said that you can accomplish anything you set your mind to. I also thought your proposal to your wife was very beautiful.—A (Wilson Hall)

Here are some notes from primary and middle school teachers:

Dr. Hickey, I wish you could have heard the cheer this morning when the grade six class read and listened to the blog and we realized that you have indeed stood at the top of Mt. Everest! What an accomplishment.—Anonymous (St. Mary's)

Dear Dr. Hickey, I'm so glad that I waited to write you until after our final Everest activity. As I had told you earlier, two teams (200 students) had worked for several weeks on an Everest unit of study. After your talk, our final summit was a climb to King's Pinnacle at Crowder's Mountain. Of the more than 150 students who went, only one student and one parent did not make it to the top. A few students were overweight, and they made it. Many students moaned and complained all the way up, but you would have been delighted to hear their comments: "If Dr. Hickey could make it up Everest, I can do this." The look on their faces and their comments were priceless when they did, indeed, reach their summit.—JP (Saluda Trail Middle School)

Dear Dr. Hickey, Wow, what a fantastic opportunity for our 5th and 6th grade students. They were mesmerized by your presentation as was I … and think your message is one everyone should hear.—KL (Wilson Hall)

Mentoring Students

Guides on the mountains are worth their weight in gold, as are mentors in nursing. The guides for students are their professors in the classroom and their clinical instructors in the hospitals, whereas our mentors as nurses are the educators and veteran nurses in the work setting. Mentoring is a two-way street: we should seek mentors to guide us and then "pay it forward" by becoming mentors for those needing guidance.

MyEverest Blog

Here are some notes from University of South Carolina nursing students:

Dr. Hickey, Congratulations on your summit! Thanks for what you are trying to do for the nursing profession as well as being an EX-CELLENT professor!—GJ

Dr. Hickey, I'm so proud of you! I can imagine how proud everyone else is of your accomplishment as well. You've always been an inspiration to me and now this just makes me want to ... do something... probably just start marathoning again. I'll let you climb the mountains!—AC

Dr. Hickey, Seeing you reach your goal certainly encourages me that I can reach my more modest summit (getting through this program). You certainly are an inspiration.—CB

Dr. Hickey, It's been great to be able to follow your trek and to know that you are now safely back at base camp, having accomplished your goal! Thanks again for your commitment to the nursing profession and for setting up the Summit Scholarship. We know that goal will be reached, too.—AW

Dr. Hickey, I'm so glad to hear that you made the descent! I'm so proud of your work that you've done. You are a great role model for nurses and prospective nurses across the nation and world. Congratulations!—AH

Congratulations. You are an inspiration to all! You definitely live life all the way! AWESOME! Thanks for representing nurses, the gamecocks, and world travelers everywhere so well. You're awesome and we are proud of you. Way to Go, Professor Hickey!—AM

Recruiting

Historically, efforts to bring new students into our profession were directed not only at high schools, but also at grade schools. As nurses, we are the best ambassadors for our profession, and I imagine that most of us have visited these schools, because what better way is there to recruit than to have the mother or father of a student speak to a class about his or her passion for nursing? However, as times change and job stability becomes questionable in many industries, there has been a very noticeable shift of second-career students into nursing, as well as students changing their major to nursing. Those interested in nursing meet nurses in the community and ask about job security, the potential for growth, and financial stability. Additionally, nurses extend themselves to promote the profession by targeting those people they feel would be great additions—and those people are found everywhere.

MyEverest Blog

My wish for you is that you can get back home to Carol ASAP and after a well deserved rest then you can start speaking about your wonderful accomplishment not only for your own self-satisfaction but also to bring awareness of the need for recruiting competent and enthusiastic people to take over the nursing profession when the nurses in our age group retire etc.

Although I have always enjoyed being a nurse the day to day grind sometimes takes a toll on my enthusiasm however, I too want to see the best come into this profession and realize just how important a calling the work can be. I find myself trying to talk people sometimes the young woman taking my order at the deli, a check-out clerk, patients etc.... into to studying to be a nurse.—SD

Create a Shared Vision

As leaders, we need to describe to others the kind of future that we can create together, and in doing so we will show others how their interest can be fulfilled by a common vision. We need to clearly communicate a positive and hopeful outlook, because this will help engage those who need direction. The vision could be something as simple as developing better communication skills in order to minimize mistakes, or confronting issues in the clinical setting.

MyEverest Blog

Pat, we are so very proud of you. Take care and we are cheering for you big time this week. The weather here is lovely but still very dry. We have many pretty flowers and singing birds reminding me of the marvelous glories of the world from SC to Mt. Everest. Have a good rest and be safe. Thank you for your efforts to raise awareness of the needs for Nursing Education.—RS, College of Nursing at USC

Challenge the Status Quo

I love to challenge the status quo… in a good way! I believe that we should always look for ways to improve and innovate, experiment and take risks, and always ask, "What can we learn?" when things don't go as expected. As a new nurse in orientation in the operating room, I would constantly ask questions regarding why we did things the way we did. I never accepted the standard response of, "We do things like this because it is the way that we have always done things." My interpretation of this response was that people may not understand the rationale for why they were doing something, even though they may be doing it the correct way. My polite resistance to accepting the way things were done, without an in-depth explanation, irritated those mentoring me in this new environment. However, over time this eagerness to know the "whys" behind all of our actions led to my position as creator of policies and procedures, and eventually to a management position.

MyEverest Blog

Oh My Gosh! I'm soooo excited for you. The FIRST nurse! It's so awesome. I'm just so proud for you for this grand accomplishment and know there will be many spin-off goals & rewards from this monumental journey. It touches my heart that along with your success you are serving others. That's the real beauty, Pat.—JO

Free Others to Act

As a leader, I always told my staff that I wanted work to be fun, and my two primary expectations were that they work as hard as I did and develop a level of respect for one another. I typically would encourage my staff to participate in planning actions that involved them and in doing so would give them the freedom to make their own decisions. By creating this atmosphere of mutual respect and trust, my staff felt empowered to work on assignments and projects. If we want to set people up to succeed, we need to give them the resources and power/flexibility that will enable them to do well. As a new director of quality improvement, I was given the task of developing a "bloodless medicine program" at my facility. Without the support of my administration, I would not have been able to orchestrate this hospital-wide program because the planning involved everyone from staff to upper administration, as well as the community at large. I was able to move forward, unhindered, with support from above and below.

Encourage the Heart

Have you ever stopped to think of your impact on others? Do you build people up and help them to succeed? Do you write notes of praise? How often do you smile? Do you touch people both physically and emotionally? How well do you really get to know people? This is all so easy to do, but done by so few! Why does there have to be so much negativity associated with our jobs and the negative connotations of catching people doing something wrong? Why is it that we have more negative notes in our personnel files than we do positive notes? Why is it that we feel the need to "write someone up" for a questionable action, as opposed to writing them up for doing something good? I believe that we need to do a much better job of praising people for a job well done and catching people doing things right. When project milestones were met, I always made it a practice to celebrate with rewards ranging from pizza parties to allowing staff to go home early, or when possible taking an extra day off for a job well done. I like to link rewards to achievements, because that makes work much more meaningful.

I pride myself on writing thank you notes to those who have gone out of their way to help or make a difference—and guess what, it takes very little effort! It's as easy as typing a letter, scribbling a note, and/or placing a phone call. The ripple effects of this tiny, positive gesture are huge. Employees will go out of their way and put forth a better effort for a leader who praises them for a job well done than they will for one who constantly berates them for poor performance.

MyEverest Blog

Amazing! Amazing! I don't know you, but I am proud of you! Many heartfelt congratulations! Your journey will inspire so many good things in the world.—SS

Model the Way

As leaders, we need to be able to "walk the walk" if we "talk the talk," because we need to lead by example. To do so, we need to be clear about our values and beliefs and then make certain that people adhere to those agreed-upon values. Being consistent in practicing what we preach is vitally important, because we are scrutinized not only by our peers, but, most importantly, by our patients. Sometimes being good isn't aiming high enough in life, and therefore we must strive for excellence. We need to bring the same commitment to excellence to whatever we do, whether as a leader or team player.

I spent the summer of 2008 working in a program that trained student nurses to develop the basic fundamental skills of nursing such as bed baths, vital signs, Accuchecks, and so forth. In this hospital-based program, I was able to model the way for my students as we engaged in basic patient care on a daily basis. The rewards were many, but most important for me was the opportunity to lead by example and in doing so "walk the walk" of nursing. This summer of fun has endeared me to my students and for them has reinforced the importance of practicing what you preach.

I always advise my students to seek role models and to take all of the positives from each role model to help mold their own persona as a future nurse. I encourage them to look for the passion in their role models, and I challenge the students to be passionate about something, anything! As role models, we need to be approachable and available to channel the commitment of our followers.

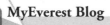

MyEverest Blog

I was in downtown Denver today (and past 3 days) experiencing positive vibes from fellow nurses and administrators who work in ambulatory surgery settings. All of them acknowledge the nursing shortage and the impact to them (having to train people into OR technique since they can no longer "steal" from the main OR staff—it is getting very short!). Who will take care of us as we age?! Your scholarship is so important, as are the other funds that are working toward training nurses. Your efforts to reach the summit will make a difference in voicing the need for more nurses and the value of nursing (differentiating our talents from the other healthcare professions—a different sort of passion, huh?!).—BD

My Climbs on the Mountains

Our legacy on the mountains as climbers is to be good stewards of the resources and to protect and preserve nature. The mountains are pristine environments of untouched nature and should be left intact as a testament to their beauty. Unfortunately, over the years there has been a lack of controls and even fewer regulations on the mountains. The maintenance of these environments has been left up to the moral character of the climbers and their support teams. As a result, there has been scarring of those mountain environments through the reckless abandonment of trash and unwanted supplies. **Mt. Everest** was the biggest victim, because for years stockpiles of empty oxygen tanks, old tents, and cached supplies littered the landscape. More recently there has been an effort to police our sport as climber after climber has contributed to the cleaning of the mountains. On my recent climb of **Mt. Everest**, I was able to witness this practice: both climbers and Sherpas were diligent about keeping the mountain clean, and each carried tanks and refuse down the hill. More and more, we are packing it in and then packing it out.

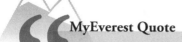

MyEverest Quote

"On a long journey even a straw weighs heavy."—Spanish Proverb

On **Mt. McKinley** in Alaska, to avoid contaminating the mountain with body waste, we drew straws among the climbers to see who would have the responsibility of carrying a porta-potty to high camp (I got the short straw). On **Mt. Vinson** in Antarctica, we were given large plastic refuse bags, which we were to use, and carry, for our bowel movements. Through each of us contributing in our own way to keeping the mountains clean, we collectively support the old saying "take only pictures and leave only footprints."

Christmas Came Early

As each of us collectively works toward the betterment of the whole, individually we all do our own things to help as best we can. On **Mt. Everest**, I celebrated my summit and subsequently my completion of the 7 Summits by contributing to the welfare of the local Sherpas. A few hours after my arrival at Base Camp, I contacted the camp manager because I wanted to show my appreciation for the efforts of his Sherpas, and I asked him to summon the climbing Sherpas and support team to a meeting. At this meeting, I thanked all for their support and then further celebrated by giving away all of my mountaineering gear! It was like Christmas for them as I gave away Gore-Tex jackets, down mitts, plastic boots, crampons, ice ax, shirts, pants, socks, and so forth. The Sherpas were most gracious on receiving these gifts, because most had very little, yet put their lives on the line daily for us climbers. It was such a thrill for me to be able to give to these hard-working locals. I could only hope that other climbers would give extra gear away as I had done. Before my trip to Nepal, I had made a promise to Carol that this was the final of the 7 Summits and upon completion I was done with mountain climbing. I felt that it would be bad karma for me to continue to climb after I had made this promise, so I kept true to my word! Besides, I could use a break from high places, because my fear of heights had been challenged way too many times.

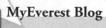

MyEverest Blog

"There are times people will touch our lives just for a fleeting moment and yet their impact will last a lifetime."—MC

Sharing the Altitude

Mt. Kilimanjaro has been considered the easiest of the 7 Summits of the World, because it is not very challenging technically, has little extreme weather with which to contend, and is a gradual climb to the top. However, the mountain is close to 20,000 feet high and, depending on the route taken, will require a 13,000–15,000-foot ascent. Also, because the terrain varies from dirt trails to rocky moonscapes to icy glaciers near the summit, the climb requires substantial cardiovascular stamina, strength, and endurance. My 2002 climb of **Mt. Kilimanjaro** was the second of the 7 Summits, but in a way it was the most memorable because I was able to climb with my wife Carol. She and I had always camped and hiked together, but until that point she had never shared my passion to challenge herself at altitude. Conditioning and training are a daily part of our lives, so there was no great need to get ourselves in any better shape than we already were; however, nothing that we could do in South Carolina could prepare us for climbing at altitude. Despite the altitude, Carol was able to make the summit, but we had to hasten our descent because she started to exhibit symptoms related to cerebral edema. For me, it was a thrill to climb with my wife because she was able to experience the elation of standing on a summit, and she was also able to better understand my continued drive to complete the 7 Summits of the World.

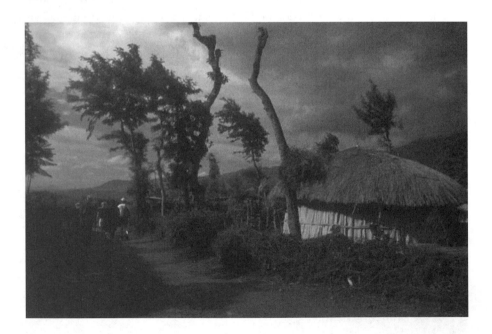

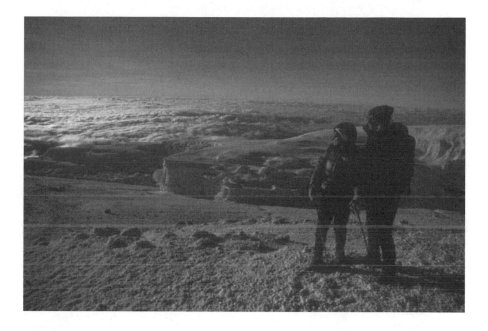

MyEverest Blog

Pat, all your friends at Richland who have been following your amazing trek take great pride in your accomplishment and cheer along with you in this momentous feat. I can't imagine what this must feel like... you have joined an elite group of world adventurers (not that you weren't already there) who have dared to stretch their personal limits and achieve greatness. Sir Edmund Hillary would be proud of you, as all of your nurse peers are. How exhilarating this is for you and for nursing!—EM

Table 8-1   Legacy Checklist

Review the following list to see how you can leave a legacy.

Realizing Your Legacy	Yes	No
Legacy		

• Have any of the following people had an influence on you to make you a better person?
  – Mom
  – Dad
  – Brothers
  – Sisters
  – Uncles
  – Aunts
  – Friends
  – Teachers		

• Feel that you have created a legacy through your contribution to:
  – Family
  – Friends
  – School
  – Charities
  – Community		

• Feel you could do more to create your own legacy		
• Feel you could do more to create the legacy of another		
• Accept that our actions as leaders contribute to our legacy		
• Realize that our actions as mentors contribute to our legacy		

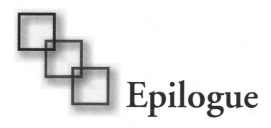

Epilogue

SURVIVAL KIT FOR NURSE MANAGERS (ITEMS INCLUDED)

Lifesavers to remind you of the strategies of success
A Band-Aid for a quick fix
A toothpick to pick the bad from the good
A paper clip to help you hold it all together
Post-Its so you can stay organized and write it all down
A string when you feel like you can't hold on any more
An eraser to erase all the bad stuff and keep the good
Tylenol for the headache that won't go away
A chocolate kiss to remind you that you are loved
Lip gloss to keep you fresh and smiling
Lotion to keep you in touch with your soft side
A tea bag to enjoy a soothing moment
And for good luck—a PayDay chocolate bar to remind you of why
you took the job!!!

—TS

Mt. Everest is not about the summit, the conquest of nature, or the conquest of other human beings. **Mt. Everest** is about commitment, goal setting, and the end of one journey and the beginning of another. **Mt. Everest** causes you to look into the faces of your fellow climbers, disheartened by fear and determined by hope, and into your own eyes in the mirror when you think that you have nothing more left in you. **Mt. Everest** is about love: for life, nature, people, and yourself. **Mt. Everest** is not about the sum-

175

mit, which is such a small piece of the mountain. Most of its beauty and wonders are experienced during the climb.

This book has been a labor of love, because writing about my life, travels, nursing, and mountain climbing has given me a rare introspective look at life. On **Mt. Everest** during my climb to Camp 4, and again on my descent off the summit, I had another introspective look at life, and death, as I saw my life flash before my eyes: severe hypothermia, dehydration, and exhaustion collectively crippled me to the point where I almost became a permanent fixture on the mountain. To see your life pass by you as you near death, and then to write in detail of those feelings, is very haunting. It was the deepest, darkest place that I have ever gone to in life, and my step over to "the other side" has changed me in ways that I never imagined.

MyEverest Blog

"If I may dare to step into the footprints of legends, I must place each step in unison with theirs and yet each step must be my own."—MC

Reflecting back on my years in the mountains, I have to say that I had "the life of Riley" because I freed myself from the routines of everyday life, spent most of the time figuring out my next meal, enjoyed panoramic views of snow-capped mountains, and heard the lonely sound of my own breath. During this journey, I explored long-suppressed thoughts hidden in the back of my brain that found their way to the surface and accompanied me through the most challenging parts. I experienced a range of emotions so intense, and so contradictory, that I could almost taste the fear, triumph, and frustration associated with my climbs. The culmination of these experiences has given me a new view of the world, humankind, loved ones, and our overall purpose in life.

The word *conquer* is used quite freely when speaking of attaining summit peaks, but how does one really conquer an inanimate object? I believe that the true conquest that occurs in the mountains is our ability to conquer ourselves. It's not a given that everyone who attempts to summit will meet their goal. Many fall short and in doing so realize failure. Most take the opportunity to face it and change, whereas others will repeat the same thing, without growing or changing.

So, which person will you be? The one to conquer yourself through facing your need to change and doing it; or will you be the one who sees the changes needed to make yourself a better person but makes the decision to stay the way you are? To help you in this decision, the steps you need to take after reading this book are to first evaluate yourself in relation to the 7 Summits of Life. To do so, review the meanings of *balance, wellness, goals, attitude, potential, success,* and *legacy* (found at the beginnings of Chapters 2–8), and compare these interpretations to yours, and then to your life. Next, you need to complete the list of proficiencies and deficiencies, or

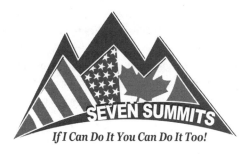

If I Can Do It You Can Do It Too!

the positives and negatives that you see in your life, by visiting the checklist found at the end of each chapter. Once completed, take the time to review the lists and see whether you have balance in your life; physical, mental, and financial wellness; established goals with timelines that you revisit often; an optimistic positive attitude; realization of your potential to do anything you want; success in life; and a legacy that will benefit others. The lists, and the evaluation, are very subjective but hopefully will cause you to take a deep internal look at yourself and your lifestyle. Conquering ourselves is the biggest challenge we will ever have; however, acknowledging the need to change is a great beginning.

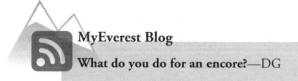

MyEverest Blog

What do you do for an encore?—DG

Once you have reviewed the 7 Summits of Life, have completed the lists at the end of each chapter, and have reviewed them according to your lifestyle, it is then time to get to work on how to make those changes. If you have achieved balance in life, but not success, then you may need to revisit your goals to establish some concrete guidelines. If you are setting your sights too high, remember the feeling of success, and work toward that goal. If wellness is an issue, work toward completion of this task by setting up a physical fitness regimen, changing your diet, reallocating funds and reprioritizing interests to assure financial stability, and getting in touch with self, family, friends, and coworkers in order to maintain mental wellness. Define your goals with timelines, categorize them, revisit them often, update them, and then delete them when you have accomplished them. Goals affect all categories of the 7 Summits of Life because you are in control of your destiny. Check your attitude often, and have family and friends validate your findings. Who better to judge our outlook on life than those who see our daily actions? And, as we all know, actions speak louder than words.

Realizing our potential requires a strong support system, because we are our own worst enemies when it comes to trying something new and challenging. Many of us have adopted a laissez-faire attitude and will not push harder because to change something that is not broken, or to do something that causes us to break into a sweat, is considered above and beyond our abilities. A support system—whether it be family, friends, or teachers—is critical to the development of our potential that sometimes lies

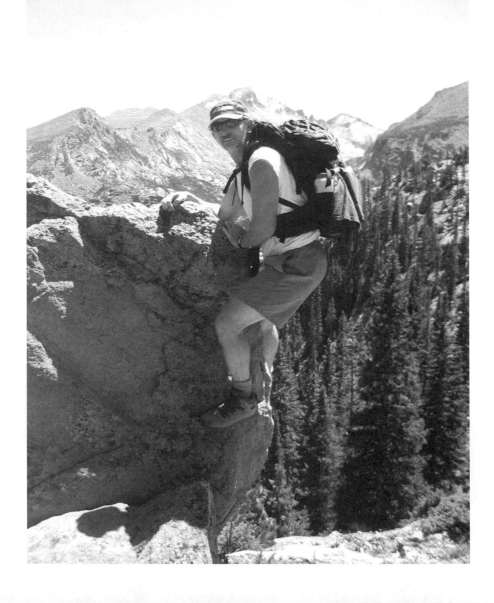

deep within and is most often dormant, just waiting to be released. Success is not about winning races or making a lot of money; success is accomplishing our goals, no matter how minimal or challenging. Successes can be many, and in small portions, and should be easily measured. And finally, create a legacy, which I believe is the most important of all the 7 Summits of Life. Just how do you create a legacy? Our legacy is built as we maneuver our way through life. It's the daily things we do such as donating to a charity, working on a committee, mentoring a student, volunteering time and skills, or simply making ourselves available to help another person in need.

You are in control of your destiny, and every decision you make affects your future—and the future of your friends, family, and coworkers. By choosing to make changes in your life, in accordance with the 7 Summits of Life, you can feel much better about yourself. What you will learn and feel can easily be transferred to those around you, because it is only natural that you would like others to enjoy life as you do. I would like to end with a quote by George Mallory that speaks to his desire to challenge himself by climbing **Mt. Everest**: "What we get from this is adventure and just sheer joy. And joy is, after all, the end of life."